Updates in Otorhinolaryngology

Edited by Georgios Giourgos

Published in London, United Kingdom

Updates in Otorhinolaryngology
http://dx.doi.org/10.5772/intechopen.1004474
Edited by Georgios Giourgos

Contributors
Anas Ibrahim, Arushi Tomar, Eleni Litsou, Elias Antoniades, Farid Alzhrani, Georgios Giourgos, Hee-Young Kim, Isra Aljazeeri, Joon Kon Kim, Reham Abdel Wakil Ibrahim, Shalini Gupta, Sharon John, Yassin Abdelsamad

First published in London, United Kingdom, 2025 by IntechOpen
IntechOpen is the global imprint of INTECHOPEN LIMITED, registered in England and Wales, registration number: 11086078, 167-169 Great Portland Street, London, W1W 5PF, United Kingdom

For EU product safety concerns: IN TECH d.o.o., Prolaz Marije Krucifikse Kozulić 3, 51000 Rijeka, Croatia, info@intechopen.com or visit our website at intechopen.com.

British Library Cataloguing-in-Publication Data
A catalogue record for this book is available from the British Library

Updates in Otorhinolaryngology
Edited by Georgios Giourgos
p. cm.
Print ISBN 978-1-83634-008-9
Online ISBN 978-1-83634-007-2
eBook (PDF) ISBN 978-1-83634-009-6

Meet the editor

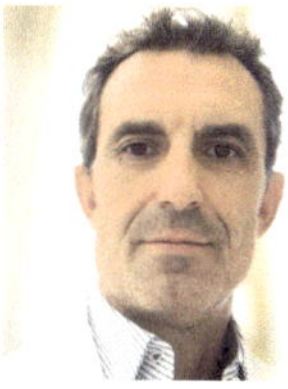

Georgios Giourgos, MD, Ph.D., is a specialist in Otorhinolaryngology-Head and Neck Surgery at the ORL Unit of ASST "Papa Giovanni XXIII" in Bergamo, holding a High Specialization position since 2022. He graduated with top honors in Medicine and Surgery in 2003, specialized in ENT with distinction in 2009, and earned a Ph. D. in Experimental Surgery and Microsurgery in 2012. With over 2,300 surgical procedures performed—more than 1,700 as the lead surgeon, he concentrates his expertise on skull base, neck and thyroid surgery, and paranasal sinus disorders. He has authored numerous scientific publications and is an active member of international scientific societies. He frequently participates in conferences and training courses as a lecturer and speaker.

Contents

Preface

Welcome to the evolving landscape of otorhinolaryngology, where each discovery helps us better understand the delicate connections between the ear, nose, and throat. The field of otorhinolaryngology has seen tremendous growth over the past few decades, thanks to the relentless efforts of researchers, clinicians, and surgeons dedicated to improving patient care.

Written by well-known authors, this book aims to provide a comprehensive overview of many recent developments in diagnosing and treating ear, nose, and throat (ENT) disorders. We delve into various topics, including auditory pathologies, nasal and sinus diseases, oropharyngeal and laryngeal conditions. Each chapter is written to offer the reader an in-depth understanding of the underlying pathophysiology, clinical presentation, and current therapeutic approaches.

One of the significant advancements in otorhinolaryngology is the advent of minimally invasive surgical techniques. Procedures such as endoscopic sinus surgery and endolaryngeal endoscopic-microscopic techniques have revolutionized how we approach ENT surgeries, reducing patient morbidity and enhancing recovery times. Furthermore, integrating cutting-edge technology like image-guided surgery and intraoperative neural monitoring has significantly improved surgical precision and patient safety.

Management of temporal bone fractures involves a multidisciplinary approach to address potential complications such as hearing loss, facial nerve injury, and cerebrospinal fluid (CSF) leaks. Initial assessment includes a high-resolution CT scan to delineate the fracture and identify any otic capsule or facial nerve canal involvement. Treatment may involve conservative measures like observation and head elevation for CSF leaks or surgical intervention for severe cases, such as facial nerve decompression or ossicular chain reconstruction.

Identifying the human papillomavirus (HPV) as a significant factor in the development of many oropharyngeal cancers has led to the inclusion of specific HPV testing as part of the diagnostic process. Implementing molecular biomarkers and liquid biopsy techniques are emerging as promising tools for early and non-invasive diagnosis, offering new opportunities for disease monitoring and personalized therapies. These advancements, alongside advanced imaging techniques and an increased understanding of the molecular characteristics of oropharyngeal carcinoma, are revolutionizing the diagnostic and therapeutic approach to this disease.

In the realm of auditory disorders, the development of implanted devices has transformed the lives of individuals with severe hearing loss. Vibrant Soundbridge ear implants are innovative devices designed to improve hearing for individuals with sensorineural hearing loss. Unlike traditional hearing aids, which amplify sound, the Vibrant Soundbridge directly stimulates the middle ear structures. This results in clearer and more natural sound perception. Additionally, advances in genetic research have paved the way for personalized medicine, offering new hope for patients with hereditary hearing loss.

This book is a testament to the relentless pursuit of knowledge and excellence in otorhinolaryngology. We hope this work will serve as a valuable resource for practitioners, researchers, and students alike, inspiring them to continue exploring the frontiers of this dynamic field.

Georgios Giourgos, MD, PhD
Otorhinolaryngology Clinic,
ASST "Papa Giovanni XXIII",
Bergamo, Italy

Chapter 1

Endoscopic Surgeries for Benign Vocal Fold Pathology: Phonomicrosurgical Voice Procedures

Reham Abdel Wakil Ibrahim

Abstract

The field of endoscopic surgeries of the vocal fold is continuously evolving. The advances in imaging and documentation of the vocal fold have rendered a paradigm shift in laryngeal micro-surgical techniques. Understanding the anatomy and physiology as well as the pathology of different vocal fold pathological conditions is of utmost importance to the laryngeal surgeon. Also, acknowledgment of the nonsurgical treatment modalities provides the basics for a better approach to vocal fold pathologies. This chapter will enclose: the basic anatomical and physiological background of the vocal fold, a brief description of different vocal fold pathologies, essential endoscopic surgical information for vocal fold surgery, and crucial information about the indications, timing, and steps of vocal fold surgeries.

Keywords: phonation, mucosa, lamina propria, phonomicrosurgery, immobility, injection, laryngoplasty, denervation

1. Introduction

Endoscopic surgeries of the vocal fold achieve the elimination of pathological structural changes of the vocal folds and at the same time permit the preservation and restoration of the pliability of the vocal fold mucosa and vibratory characteristics. Endoscopic surgeries for voice disorders have much evolved over the past 20 years, so this chapter aims to provide the basis for endoscopic surgeries of the vocal fold in addition to the recent surgical trends for the management of different voice disorders. Knowledge of the basis of vocal fold pathology is imperative for a successful vocal fold surgery; therefore, this chapter is prepared to bring together the essential anatomy and pathology of different vocal fold pathologies, the indications and contraindications of vocal fold endoscopic surgeries, as well as the key points and pitfalls of endoscopic surgeries of the vocal fold.

2. Anatomical and physiological background

2.1 Laryngeal cartilages

- *Hyoid bone:* The laryngeal framework comprises nine cartilages interconnected with ligaments and membranes. The hyoid bone is not included within the laryngeal cartilage; however, it is crucial for some vocal fold injection procedures. It is a horseshoe-shaped bone situated in the anterior midline of the neck and gives an attachment to a variety of muscles in the mouth floor and some of the extrinsic laryngeal muscles. It is connected to the larynx by the thyrohyoid membrane.

- *Thyroid cartilage:* It is the largest of the laryngeal cartilages, which is composed of two rectangular laminae that are incompletely fused anteriorly in the midline forming the superior thyroid notch. Superior and inferior cornua are attached to each lamina posterior; the superior one gives an attachment to the greater horn of the hyoid bone via the thyrohyoid membrane, whereas the inferior cornu articulates with the cricoid cartilage, forming the cricothyroid joint. The thyroid cartilage protects the vocal folds that are attached near to its lower border, not at its midpoint, as it's wrongly assumed; this is important for the correct placement of the thyroid window in vocal fold medialization thyroplasty.

- *Cricoid cartilage:* It is a signet ring-shaped cartilage that sits dorsally inferior to the thyroid cartilage. It gives an attachment to the arytenoid cartilage.

- *Arytenoid cartilages:* They are paired pyramidal cartilages that lie on the dorsal aspect of the larynx articulating to the cricoid cartilage inferiorly. The vocal process (medially) and the muscular process (laterally) emanate from each arytenoid cartilage. These processes give attachments to the vocal ligament and intrinsic muscles of the larynx, respectively.

- *Epiglottis:* Fibro-elastic cartilage attached to the inner surface of the thyroid cartilage. It is displaced posteriorly by the hyolaryngeal excursion and tongue base contraction to cover the laryngeal inlet, thus aiding in airway protection during swallowing.

- *Cuneiform and corniculate cartilages*: They are small, paired cartilages that support the opening of the laryngeal vestibule both dorsally and laterally by firming the aryepiglotic folds [1, 2].

2.2 Laryngeal joints

The laryngeal cartilages are joined by two sets of synovial joints. One pair formed from the articulation of the inferior cornu of the thyroid cartilage and the cricoid cartilage articulatory facet; the cricothyroid joint has two major actions, an anteroposterior sliding and rotatory movements of the thyroid cartilage about the cricoid cartilage, thus allowing the cricoid cartilage to discrete from or approximate to the thyroid cartilage. The cricoarytenoid joint resembles a shallow ball and socket, thus allowing rotatory movement of the whole arytenoid not just the vocal process.

Consequently, the vocal folds move in a three-dimensional plane. This is of particular importance in cases of UVFP, where there might be some height differences between the vocal folds, and in such instances, the full coaptation of the vocal fold edges might not be achieved by injection medialization alone (**Figures 1** and **2**) [3, 4].

2.3 Laryngeal muscles

1. *Intrinsic muscles:* These muscles are concerned with changing the position, shape, and length of the vocal folds. They are classified functionally into: adductors (thyroarytenoid, lateral cricoarytenoid, and interarytenoid), abductors (posterior cricoarytenoid), sphincters (oblique arytenoid and aryepiglottic), and tensors (cricothyroid).

2. *Extrinsic muscles:* They are responsible for movement of the hyoid bone, hence movement of the larynx within the neck and also providing additional stabilization of the larynx. They include the infrahyoid muscles (sternohyoid, omohyoid, thyrohyoid, sternothyroid) and suprahyoid muscles (stylohyoid, mylohyoid, geniohyoid, digastric) [2].

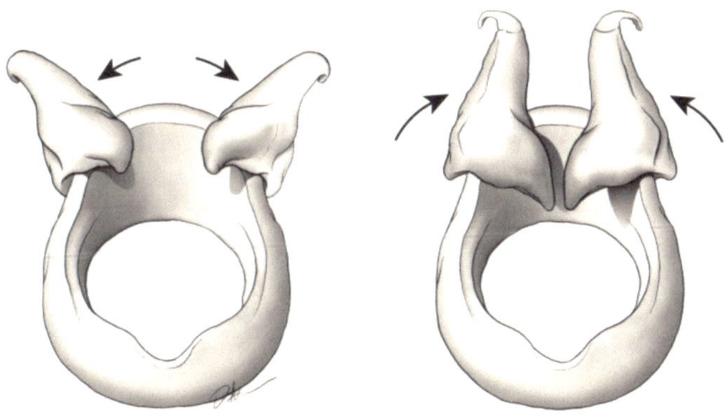

Figure 1.
Cricoarytenoid joint movement where there is a rotation of the vocal process of the arytenoid cartilage outward (laterally and postero-superiorly) and inward (medially and antero-inferiorly) causing abduction and adduction of the vocal folds, respectively (Bryant et al. [3]).

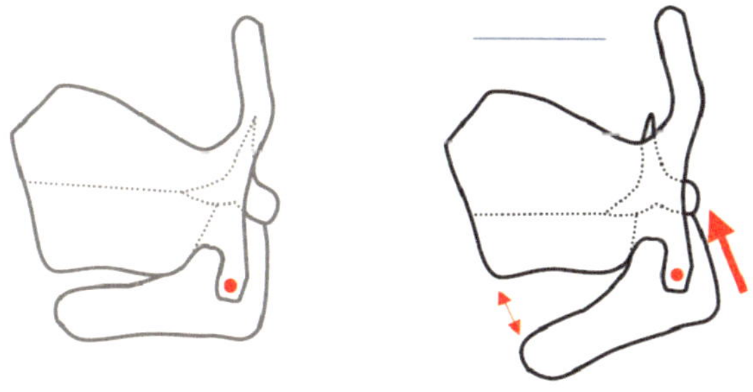

Figure 2.
Cricothyroid joint movement by which there is tilting of the anterior aspect of the cricoid cartilage upward, thus decreasing the anterior space between the thyroid cartilage inferior border and cricoid cartilage upper border Ref. [4].

2.4 Laryngeal folds and membranes

The fibroelastic tissue provides the larynx support during mechanical movements. They can be divided into two categories: extrinsic and intrinsic ligaments and membranes. The extrinsic ligaments surrounding the larynx are the thyrohyoid membrane and hyoepiglottic and cricotracheal ligaments. The thyrohyoid membrane connects the anterior aspect of the thyroid cartilage with the hyoid bone superiorly. The hyoepiglottic and cricotracheal ligaments join the hyoid bone superiorly and the trachea inferiorly. The quadrangular membrane and cricothyroid ligament support the larynx intrinsically and function as barriers preventing the spread of laryngeal malignancy. The cricothyroid ligament includes both the cricothyroid membrane and conus elasticus. The former connects the cricoid and thyroid cartilages, whereas the later, sometimes also called the lateral cricothyroid ligament, arises along the superior border of the cricoid cartilage and extends laterally and superiorly to attach to the anterior commissure and vocal process [2].

2.5 Innervation and blood supply

The vagus (cranial nerve X) nerve gives sensory and motor innervation to the larynx via the superior and recurrent laryngeal nerves (RLN). The superior laryngeal nerve (SNL) provides sensory innervation to the supraglottic and glottis larynx and motor innervation to the cricothyroid muscle. Recently, some studies have postulated that the ventricularis muscle (superior part of the thyroarytenoid muscle in the ventricular fold) may possess some motor innervation from the SLN, which may justify the movement of the ventricular fold in RLN injury. The recurrent laryngeal nerve provides motor innervation to the intrinsic laryngeal muscles, except the cricothyroid and sensory innervation to the glottis and subglottic laryngeal mucosa. Nevertheless, it must be kept in mind that in unilateral recurrent laryngeal nerve injury, the interarytenoid muscle is an unpaired muscle that will still receive input from the contralateral RLN; hence, there may be some adductory movement of the paralyzed vocal fold.

The superior and inferior laryngeal arteries provide arterial supply to the larynx, and the venous supply follows the same path [2].

2.6 Surgical anatomy of the vocal fold

The vocal fold is a versatile multilayered structure. It is composed of the following layers: squamous epithelium; lamina propria which includes three layers: superficial (SLP), intermediate, and deep layers (the intermediate and deep lamina propria form the vocal ligament); and the vocalis muscle. The lamina propria contains extracellular matrix produced by fibroblasts and has varying degrees of elasticity escalating from the deep to superficial layers owing to the amount of elastin and collagen fibers where elastic fibers decrease and collagen fibers increase with each descending layer. The superficial lamina propria is referred to as the Reinke's space, which has a thickness of about 0.3 mm. The Reinke's space is the region that vibrates most extensively during phonation, and it is the potential area for fluid accumulation in cases of Reinke's edema. It has to be put in mind that the vocal fold has three surfaces, which are designated as the three lips: upper, middle, and lower lips, giving it the virtue of three-dimensional vibratory function, which appears in cross-sectional views (**Figure 3**) [5].

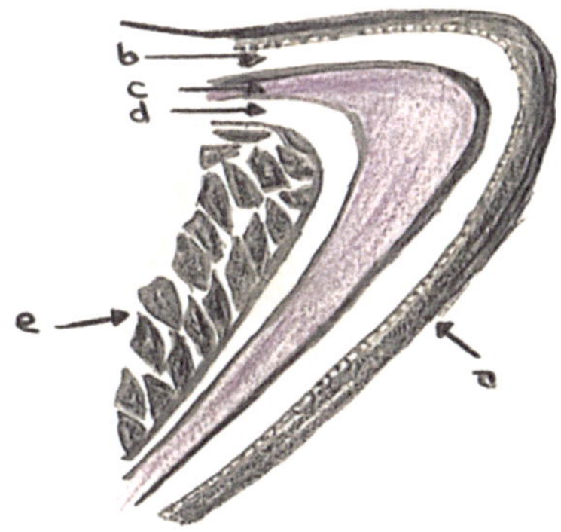

Figure 3.
Layer structure of the vocal fold. a: epithelial layer, b: superficial layer of the lamina propria, c: intermediate layer, d: deep layer, and e: vocalis muscle.

2.7 Laryngeal physiology

The larynx has four basic functions: airway protection, respiration, swallowing (elevation with the hyoid bone to aid swallowing), and phonation. Phonation is an extremely specialized function that entails a high level of cortical support signaling the activity of the thyroarytenoid and lateral cricoarytenoid muscles accompanied by movement of the diaphragm and abdominal muscles. Phonation begins by inhalation and ensuing glottis closure. Accordingly, air pressure is built up beneath the vocal folds (subglottic air pressure), which pushes the vocal folds to open (opening phase). Approximation of the edges of the vocal fold follows, and air passes between the vocal folds, resulting in the formation of the mucosal wave; hereby, the loose pliable vocal fold mucosa moves over the stiff vocalis muscle and vocal ligament (body-cover complex). This movement starts at the infraglottic area and then is transmitted to the free edge and propagated laterally over the superior surface of the vocal fold. This sequence of events is called the glottis cycle [2].

3. Evaluation of vocal fold pathology

Functional assessment of vocal fold pathology is crucial to determine the effect of any treatment of vocal fold disorder either by surgical or medical treatment. Also, it permits comparisons of different investigational procedures. The evaluation basically consists of the following parameters:

1. Patient interview, history taking, and quality of life questionnaires

2. *Auditory perceptual assessment:* The term “Dysphonia” is used to describe any deviant voice quality. Hoarseness of voice is rather a non-specific term describing a noticeable noise component in the voice. There are a variety of scales used to subjectively analyze the perceived dysphonia such as GRBAS scale [6] where G represents the overall grade of dysphonia, R reflects the subjective

impression of the voice irregularity, B is the breathiness that results from air leakage occurring with glottis insufficiency, A is the voice asthenia and weakness, and S represents the strained voice quality. Other scales include the (CAPE-V) Consensus Auditory-Perceptual- Evaluation- Voice [7] and RBH scale by Refs. [6, 8–11].

3. *Acoustic analysis and aerodynamic measure:* They both provide an objective evaluation of the voice function.

4. *Videostroboscopic examination:* Stroboscopy is based on the idea of providing a rapid succession of light flashes to illuminate a moving object. The frequency of these light flashes is appropriate to the frequency of the moving object, and since the human eye is only able to perceive a moving object frequency of maximally 20 Hz, stroboscopy allows slow-motion visualization of vocal fold vibration, in other words, a pseudo motion representation. Utilizing laryngostroboscopy, the following characteristics of the vibratory cycle are evaluated; pattern and duration of vocal fold closure, presence or absence of mucosal wave, symmetry and amplitude of vocal fold vibration, phonatory waste, and periodicity and phase differences of the vocal fold vibratory cycle.

5. *Rigid and flexible laryngoscopy:* The rigid laryngoscopy entails a metal rod ranging from 15 to 25 cm in length. The light is reflected by a mirror at the tip of the endoscope. There are two types of rigid laryngoscopy, 70–90°, depending on the angle of light reflection. The flexible laryngoscope is about 40 cm in length and of varying diameters reaching down to 0.2 mm to be suitable to use in pediatrics [6].

4. Benign lesions of the vocal fold

They are non-malignant lesions occurring almost always at the midmembranous portion of the vocal fold as it is the area of the most extensive vibration, hence liable to be injured from excessive mechanical trauma during phonation, resulting in alteration of the superficial lamina propria and occasionally the basement membrane zone of the surface epithelium. They share common predisposing factors, namely voice abuse or misuse, smoking, chronic infection of the upper respiratory tract (URTI), gastro-esophageal reflux (GERD), and nasal allergy. These lesions are among the most common voice disorders, and unfortunately, they can lead to a significant handicap, especially for professional voice users. They include: vocal fold nodules, cysts, polyps, Reinke's edema, contact granuloma of the vocal process, and bamboo nodes.

4.1 Vocal fold nodules

Bilateral small (< 3 mm in size) symmetrical swellings on the free edges of the vocal fold classically at the junction between the anterior and middle thirds of the vocal fold, arising mainly in the superficial layer of lamina propria and basement membrane zone of the surface epithelium. It occurs primarily in adult females and both genders in children (a disease of high-pitched voice). Videostroboscopy reveals almost normal mucosal waves yet with a characteristic hour-glass phonatory waste. The first line of management is voice therapy, to eliminate the maladaptive vocal behavior. Intralesional steroid injection demonstrates significant improvement especially when the patient's working conditions require rapid recovery of the voice problem. Surgical excision is considered only in cases where the conventional non-surgical treatment has failed and for cases with hard fibrotic nodules [12].

4.2 Vocal fold cysts

Benign lesions are situated in the midmembranous vocal fold embedded in the subepithelial layer. Two types are recognized: epidermoid and mucous retention cyst. The affected vocal fold appears bulged with occasional vascular atresia on the mucosal surface. Stroboscopic examination reveals abnormal mucosal waves overlying the region of the cyst. Conservative treatment as voice rest and voice therapy are rarely beneficial alone. Although intralesional steroid injection have demonstrated some remission of the size of the cyst, surgical excision is likely the treatment of choice [13].

4.3 Vocal fold polyps

These are lesions, arising at the midmembranous portion of the vocal fold. It has various morphological types including gelatinous, which is likely sessile with a broad base; hemorrhagic, which is usually situated on the upper surface of the vocal fold; hyaline; and fibrous polyps. Phonotrauma is the primary predisposing factor of vocal fold polyp; however, other etiologies such as smoking, nasal obstruction, occupational exposure, and gastroesophageal reflux also exist. On laryngostroboscopy, they appear as sessile or pedunculated growths with reduced or absent mucosal waves depending on the size of the lesion; irregular vocal fold vibration and incomplete glottis closure can also be noticed. Traditionally, they are treated by surgical excision. However, other treatment modalities are available, namely, conservative medical treatment with corticosteroid, which is indicated mainly for small polyps. Vocal fold steroid injection has been effective in complete resolution of small-sized polyps; nevertheless, the results were associated with a high rate of recurrence due to the absorption of steroids from the injection sites. Voice therapy should be prioritized for all cases to adjust the faulty vocal behavior preferably to be done before and after surgical excision [13, 14].

4.4 Reinke's edema (polypoid corditis)

Chronic benign lesion of the vocal fold entails diffuse swelling of the superficial lamina propria of the vocal fold due to fluid accumulation in Reinke's space. Smoking is the primary predisposing factor (97%); very often voice abuse and misuse are associated with its occurrence, and sometimes also GERD is a contributing factor. Clinically, it is associated mainly with a lowering of the fundamental frequency and a resultant low-pitched voice. Also, vocal fatigue and, in severe cases, airway obstruction might be encountered. Laryngostroboscopy shows unilateral or bilateral fusiform swelling of the vocal folds with increased amplitude and propagation of the mucosal wave. Stern recommendation to quit smoking and behavior modification voice therapy should be prioritized before surgical management. Medical treatment including antireflux medication is beneficial before surgery to allow re-epithelization of the vocal fold. Hyalurinidaze injection to counteract the heightening effect of hyaluronic acid in the superficial lamina propria has proven its efficiency. Mild cases of Reinke's edema have undergone complete remission after local steroid injection. However, patients may need multiple injections, and the recurrence rate is somewhat high [15, 16].

4.5 Contact granuloma

Benign granulomatous lesion arises at the medial surface of the vocal process of the arytenoid cartilage. Hard glottal attack with hyperadduction forces of the arytenoid cartilages, laryngopharyngeal reflux, and abnormal vocal behavior are commonly predisposing factors. It also may be associated with smoking and frequent upper respiratory tract infections. Treatment is mainly conservative and includes voice therapy, antibiotics, corticosteroids, and antireflux treatment. Voice therapy aims at altering the maladaptive vocal behavior and producing easy onset phonation and decreasing the excessive adduction at the arytenoids. Botulinum toxin injection has proven its efficiency in eliminating the arytenoid cartilage hyperadduction by chemical denervation of the thyroarytenoid and lateral cricoarytenoid muscle complex. Surgical excision is only confined to cases with acute airway obstruction [13, 14].

4.6 Bamboo nodes

These are autoimmune disease-specific lesions of the vocal fold. They appear as yellowish circumscribed lesions bulging from the middle third of the vocal fold with interruption of the vibratory activity of the vocal folds on stroboscopic examination. Typically, they occur secondary to autoimmune disease such as systemic lupus erythromatosis and rheumatoid arthritis. The first line of management is systemic corticosteroids. Local injection of prednisolone 5 mg or triamcinolone 1 ml causes regression of the nodes; however, there is the incidence of recurrence; thus, repeated injection is implemented. Surgical excision via a micro flap technique along with systemic corticosteroids are indicated in refractory cases; nonetheless, postoperative scar formation might worsen the dysphonia [14].

4.7 Vocal fold vascular malformations

These are lesions resulting from enlargement or dilatation of the vocal fold vessels. They mainly result from acute vocal trauma; however, other etiologies such as GERD, URTI, anticoagulant medication, and smoking may also be involved. Different forms are identified; they may be submucosal hemorrhage, vascular ectasia, or atresia. The dilated blood vessels run parallel to the longitudinal access of the vocal fold. Videostroboscopy shows impairment of the mucosal waves. Voice therapy may be of benefit, yet surgical management is indicated in most cases [17].

5. Dysplastic lesions of the vocal fold

5.1 Vocal fold leukoplakia

These are unilateral or bilateral white patches on the vocal fold surface. They appear as single or multiple foci scattered over the vocal folds and arytenoid cartilages, histologically characterized by abnormal epithelial hypertrophy and varying degrees of hyperkeratosis. The condition tends to be recurrent with a risk of malignant transformation from 1 to 40%. Smoking, viral infection, phonotrauma, and Laryngopharyngeal reflux (LPR) are supposed to be predisposing factors. Surgical excision is the ideal treatment modality, and considering the high recurrence rate, strict follow-up is mandatory.

5.2 Vocal fold dysplasia

It is a histological diagnosis, characterized by hyperchromatism, increased nuclear-cytoplasmic ratio, and anisocytosis. The condition may be asymptomatic or the patient may suffer from varying degrees of dysphonia depending on the grade of dysplasia. Videostroboscopy reveals diffuse hyperemia, swelling, and opacity of the vocal fold mucosa with erythroplakia patches along with variable degrees of interruption of the vibratory characteristics of the superficial lamina propria. Carcinoma *in situ* is a severe form of vocal fold dysplasia where the basement membrane is kept from carcinomatous invasion. Complete surgical excision for both conditions with a cold steel instrument or CO_2 laser is the ideal treatment option followed by histopathological examination. Previous practices recommended stripping of the vocal fold mucosa; however, evidence showed that it was accompanied by a high rate of recurrence. Malignant transformation has been allegedly prevented by chemotherapeutic agents such as retinoids or selenium that have been associated with the prevention of laryngeal hyperplasia; however, recurrence was more likely to occur following discontinuation of the treatment. Also, the treatment was associated with mucocutaneous toxicity.

5.3 Vocal fold carcinoma

Squamous cell carcinoma represents 90% of glottis carcinoma, commencing at the free mucosal edge of the vocal fold and then spreading to involve other laryngeal compartments. Dysphonia is the first presenting symptom; however, other manifestations as dysphagia can occur in later stages. Laryngeal examination shows white exophytic growths and grayish or pinkish granular swelling that may be confined to part or involving the whole length of the vocal fold. Stroboscopy demonstrates fixation of the mucosal vibration progressing to complete impairment of the vocal fold mobility in advanced cases. Primarily, surgical treatment with cordectomy is indicated for early stages of glottis carcinoma, and then the treatment progresses from partial to total laryngectomy for late stages [18].

6. Surgical approach to benign lesions of the vocal fold (phonomicrosurgery)

Phonomicrosurgery refers to a group of interventions addressed to restore the normal vocal characteristics and the normal vibratory pattern of the vocal fold mucosa. Nevertheless, it has to be kept in mind that regardless of the procedure used to decrease the vocal fold mass, there is a risk of vocal fold scarring. Excessive manipulation of the vocal fold mass can hinder the healing of the mucosa. Therefore, care should be implemented to justify the timing, surgical indications, and contraindications of phonomicrosurgery and preoperative and postoperative voice care. The outcome of surgery is further influenced by the selection of the appropriate surgical technique, the experience of the surgeon, the anesthetic, and airway conditions [19].

6.1 Indications of phonosurgery

It is considered to retrieve the morphological and functional characteristics of the vocal fold provided that a significant duration of voice therapy, restriction of predisposing factors, and treatment of comorbid medical conditions have all been exhausted unless there is a huge polyp encroaching on the airway, associated with dysphagia and malignant suspicion. A further indication is establishing a full coaptation of vocal fold edges as in cases of glottis insufficiency by vocal fold medialization surgeries.

6.2 Preoperative voice care

For phonomicrosurgery especially in the treatment of benign vocal fold pathology, the following should be verified:

a. *Preoperative voice therapy:* Entailing a stern vocal hygiene with a sum of dos and don'ts such as restriction of voice abuse and misuse, avoidance of any laryngeal irritants like smoking, fumes and pollutants, and alcohol consumption. Also, excessive fluid intake. Then, various holistic approaches are encountered to alter the maladaptive vocal behavior. Voice therapy should precede the surgery and is continued for at least 1–2 months afterward.

b. *The limitation of any vocal tasks:* Especially for professional voice users for not less than 2 weeks before surgery.

c. *Treatment of concomitant medical conditions:* Such as URTI, GERD, and nasal allergy.

This is crucial because any state precipitating temporary vocal fold edema such as shouting, screaming, heavy vocal demands for singers. Also, gastroesophageal reflux, nasal allergy, and upper respiratory tract infections can lead to the removal of excess vocal fold tissue which appears potentially pathological during surgery and hinders the healing of the vocal fold mucosa. Preoperative voice therapy is essential due to its role in achieving maximum postoperative voice quality and patient's compliance and minimizing any negative psych or stress from the surgery especially for professional voice users. The holistic approaches for voice therapy are beyond the purpose of this chapter.

6.3 Preoperative anesthetic consideration

1. *Careful examination:* Including Ear, Nose, and Throat (ENT), head and neck examination to exclude physical criteria speculating difficult intubation or difficult laryngeal exposure such as retrognathia, hypertrophy of the lingual tonsils, short thick neck, and cervical spondylosis with limited neck extension.

2. *The 3-3-2 rule:* Using fingers to measure the distance between fixed points; the first "3" denotes a three-finger distance between the upper and lower teeth of an open mouth; less than this can predict trismus. The following "3" represents a three-finger distance from the anterior tip of the mandible to the anterior neck, which reflects the volume of the submandibular space. The later "2" is a two-finger measurement from the floor of the mandible to the superior thyroid notch referring to the position of the larynx in the anterior neck in comparison to the tongue base. In cases where the distance is less than two fingers, then one would assume an anterior high position of the larynx rendering difficult intubation and laryngeal exposure [20].

3. *Managing difficult intubation/laryngeal exposure:*

- Tracheostomy.
- Endotracheal intubation (ETT) via an awake flexible laryngoscopy.
- Anterior commissure laryngoscopy used for intubation and laryngeal exposure.
- Intubation, utilizing a sliding Jackson Laryngoscope and endotracheal intubation by using a stylet to guide the insertion of the ETT.
- Office-based procedure and removal of the lesion in the awake settings.

6.4 Anesthesia

Phonomicrosurgery utilizes general anesthesia and endotracheal intubation (ETT) (orotracheal) with complete muscle relaxation. The choice of the ETT is crucial; a small-sized ETT (5 or 5.5) tube is the ideal diameter to avoid injury of the vocal fold or elicit mechanical pressure on the arytenoid cartilages. Other anesthetic modes such as jet ventilation and apneic techniques, for example, transnasal humidified rapid insufflation ventilator exchange (THRIVE), can be used as alternatives to ETT particularly in lesions of the posterior third of the vocal folds (vocal process and arytenoid lesions). However, these methods provide a limited operative time.

6.5 Patient poisoning for phonomicrosurgery

Lying supine with the neck flexed on the body and the head extended on the neck. This position is achieved through using the laryngoscope, which is fastened to a suspension device. The operating microscope should coincide with the longitudinal axis of the laryngoscope, and binocular vision should be secured during the whole procedure (**Figure 4**) [19].

6.6 Surgical equipment

6.6.1 Large diameter laryngoscope

Ideally, it is the most suitable for optimal laryngeal exposure. The laryngoscope is introduced through the mouth (make sure to retract the lips and protect the teeth-by-teeth protector) passed along the ventral surface of the tongue and curved backward along the posterior pharyngeal wall (or passed underneath the ETT); once approaching the epiglottis, a slight head extension is applied, and the laryngoscope is pushed forward toward the endolarynx passing below the laryngeal surface of the epiglottis. The laryngoscope should be able to visualize the entire vocal fold retracting the ventricular folds. Special attention should be provided to avoiding retracting the vocal fold. The endoscope should be confronting the upper surface of the vocal fold (**Figure 5A** and **B**) [19].

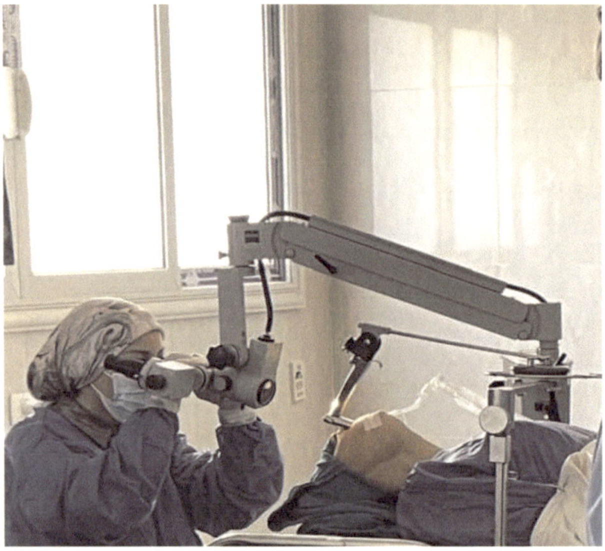

Figure 4.
Patient's position for phonmicrosurgery. Notice the neck flexed on the body and the head extension on the neck and the position of the microscope relevant to the laryngoscope.

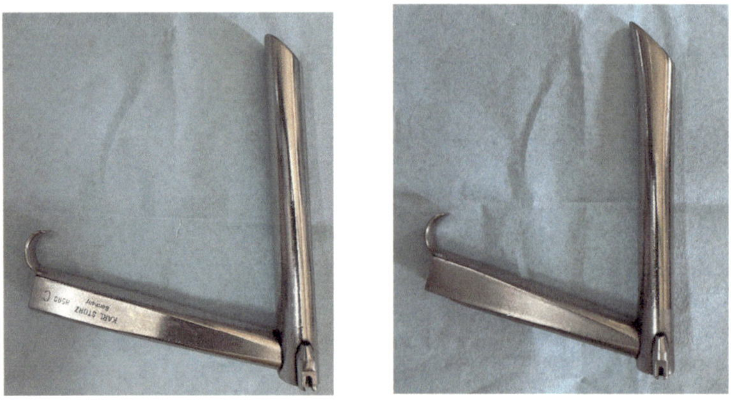

(A) (B)

Figure 5.
Operating laryngoscopes. (A) Large-bore laryngoscope, (B) Anterior commissure laryngoscope.

6.6.2 Other equipment

I.Magnification and photo documentation:

- Operating Microscope: Equipped with 400 mm lens to facilitate high magnification of the ultrastructure of the vocal fold (**Figure 4**).

- An alternative to the microscope is the rigid telescopes 0-, 30-, and 70-degrees, which allow visualization of the inferior surface of the vocal fold that cannot be visualized by the microscope.

II.Microsurgical Instruments:

- Triangular (Bouchayer) forceps; curved left, right, and straight (for anterior commissure lesions).
- Microcup forceps (1–2 mm in diameter); curved right and left.
- Microscissors; curved right and left, angled upward.
- Microlaryngeal knife (Sickle, rounded, or spear).
- Straight or curved alligator forceps
- Laryngeal microelevator and microretractor (**Figures 6–10**).

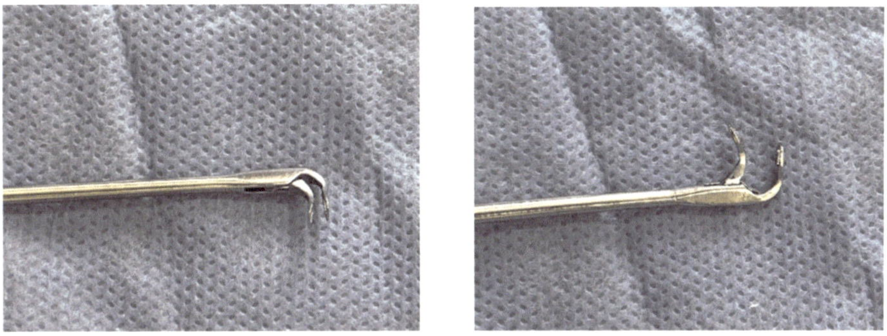

Figure 6.
Triangular forceps, curved right and left.

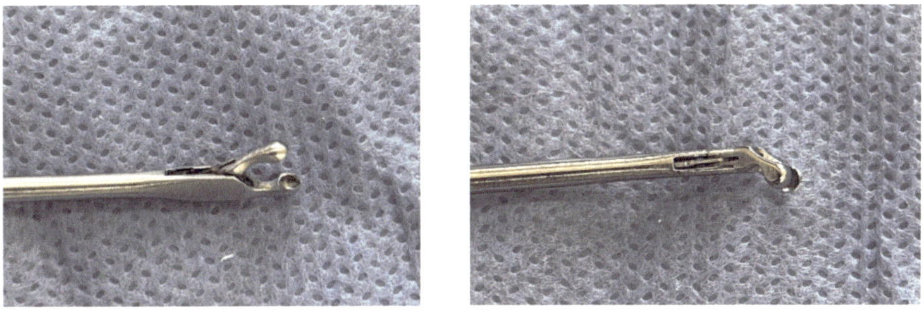

Figure 7.
Microcup forceps, straight and curved right.

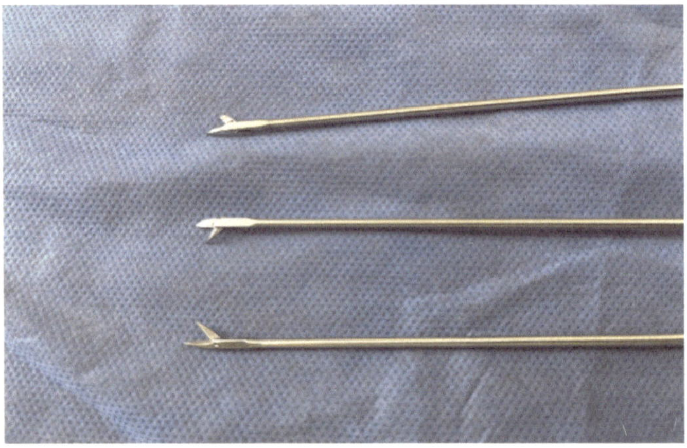

Figure 8.
Microlaryngeal scissors: Curved right, left, and straight.

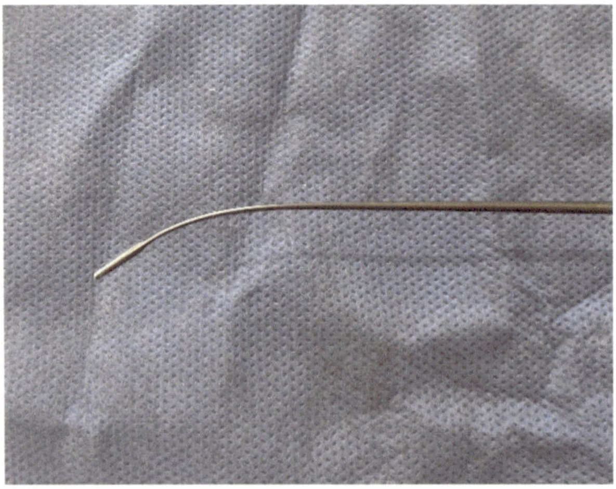

Figure 9.
Laryngeal microelevator.

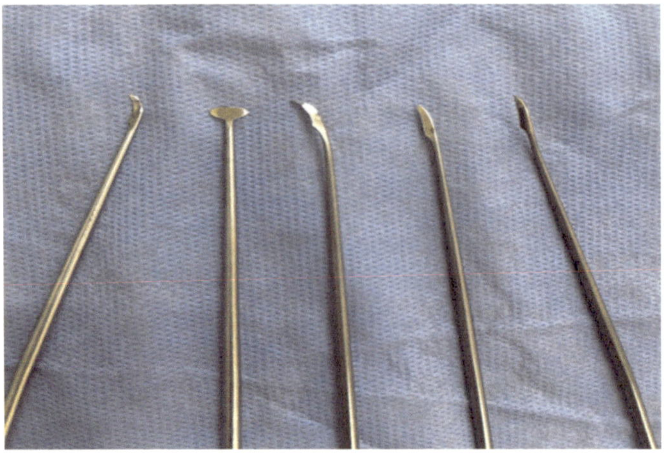

Figure 10.
Microlaryngeal knives.

7. Surgical technique

7.1 Vocal fold cyst

- An incision is made on the superior surface of the vocal fold immediately lateral to the cyst in an anterior-posterior direction with a slight extension beyond the region of the cyst (note that the incision should be superficial as possible and better to be done using the microlaryngeal knife).
- Using the microelevator with its tip directed medially to dissect the epithelial cover from the cyst wall, sometimes, the cyst wall is adherent to the epithelial cover, so care must be taken to avoid puncture of the cyst (Blunt dissection can be performed by a small cottonoid).
- Applying gentle medial traction, the dissection is continued inferiorly to separate the cyst from the vocal ligament (Note that the vocal ligament appears white with less vascularity).
- Once the dissection is completed and all attachments are freed, the cyst is excised, and the flap is reapproximated.
- If the cyst wall is punctured, grab the cyst wall and clear all the contents to avoid recurrence [19].

7.2 Vocal fold polyp

- The polyp is held by triangular forceps with the application of gentle medial traction in a perpendicular direction to the longitudinal axis of the vocal fold (Some surgeons prefer to apply an epinephrine-soaked cottonoid on the polyp for clear delineation of the base).
- Use microscissors (It is better to use one that is curved in an opposite direction to the forceps away from the vocal fold or a straight one) and cut the polyp at the junction of its base with the free edge of the vocal fold in a posterior to anterior fashion.
- Tapping the operative site with epinephrine-soaked cottonoid for several minutes and palpation of the vocal fold for any remnants that appear to be thin and atrophic or is excessive and does not function as healthy glistening vocal fold mucosa. This residual abnormal mucosa or remnants should be removed by grasping with a triangular forceps and then excision of the excess mucosa with a microscissor or remove the remnants using a 1-mm microcup forceps.
- The mentioned technique is called the truncation technique. Another technique is the microflap technique where a lateral epithelial incision is made to elevate an epithelial flap, the contents of the polyp is suctioned, and the flap is reapproximated with excision of the excess redundant unhealthy mucosa until having a straightened edge (**Figure 11**) [19].

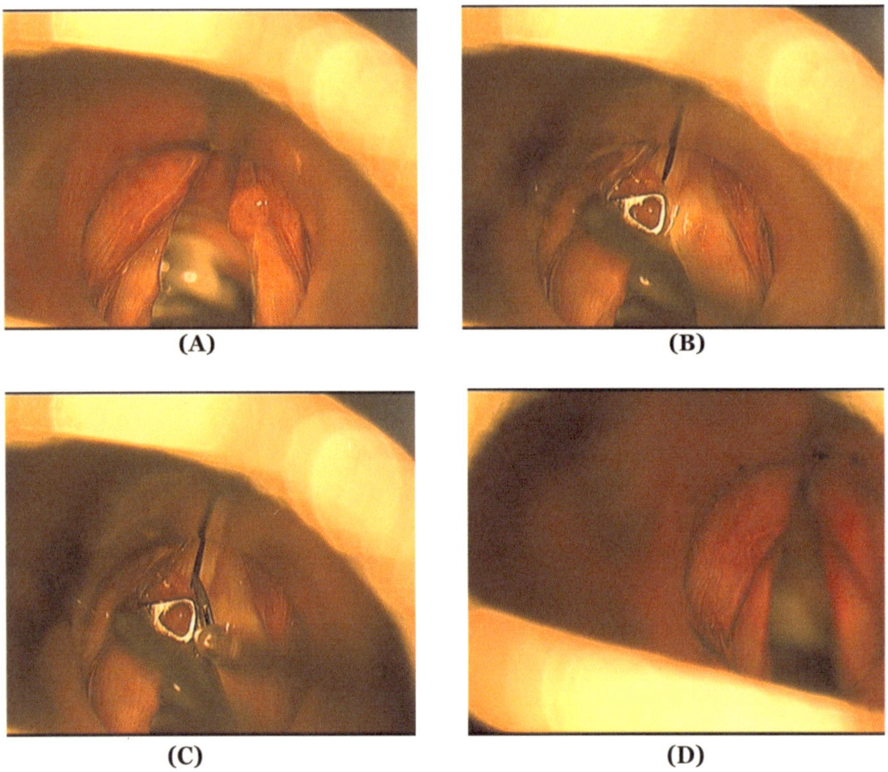

Figure 11.
Steps of excision of vocal fold pedunculated polyp by truncation technique. (A) Illustrates the preoperative direct microlaryngoscopy view, (B) grasping the polyp by triangular forceps, (C) cutting the polyp by laryngeal microscissor while applying gentle medial traction, and (D) is the immediate post excision view.

7.3 Vocal fold nodules

- They are excised with the same truncation technique as the vocal fold polyp.

7.4 Reinke's edema

- The microflap technique is the ideal approach for surgical excision where a longitudinal incision is made on the upper surface of the vocal fold just parallel to the lateral edge forming an epithelial flap, then surgical reduction in an anterior-to-posterior direction with preservation of a healthy mucosal surfaces is performed.

- Suction of the materials after retraction of the flap with a laryngeal microretractor.

- The flap is redraped, and the healthy mucosal surfaces are approximated. Sometimes in extensive cases with large defects, the two edges of the flap are sutured or glued [19].

7.5 Contact granuloma of the vocal fold

- It is best removed via jet ventilation for the anesthesia; nevertheless, an anterior position of the endotracheal tube anterior to the laryngoscope can be used for the best exposure of the posterior glottis.
- The granuloma is best gripped with curved alligator forceps in an opposite direction of the vocal fold.
- With the application of gentle medial traction, the granuloma is cut at its base with curved microscissiors in the same direction as the forceps.
- In cases of recurrent lesions, vocal fold botulinum toxin injection is done into the TA/LCA muscle complex after the surgical excision [19].

7.6 Postoperative voice rest versus voice therapy

- All patients are instructed to have an absolute voice rest ranging from 2 days to 2 weeks according to the affection of the vocal fold; this is followed by videostroboscopic examination to monitor the outcome of surgery. Voice therapy is advisable to continue for up to 1–2 months postoperatively [19].

8. Approach to Glottic insufficiency

It is a condition that refers to incomplete closure of the vocal fold hindering the full coaptation of the vocal fold edges during phonation. It's presented mainly with dysphonia, however, sometimes associated with dysphagia and risk of aspiration. Various etiological factors are involved including but not limited to vocal fold paralysis or paresis with complete immobility or partial immobility of the vocal fold. Other factors include vocal fold atrophy either local as in vocal fold tissue loss or diffuse as in presbyphonia, vocal fold sulcus or scars [21].

1. *Unilateral vocal fold paralysis (UVFP):* Surgical trauma of the recurrent laryngeal nerve as in anterior neck surgeries particularly thyroidectomy represents the most common etiology. Other factors include non-laryngeal malignancy, endotracheal intubation, or even idiopathic. Dysphonia is the primary symptom; the voice may be asthenic breathy due to air leak, gurgle-y due to secretion accumulation in the pyriform, or paralytic falsetto due to hyperfunction of the cricothyroid or extralaryngeal muscles. Dysphagia with the risk of aspiration can occur especially with high vagal injury. Videostroboscopy reveals fluttering waves and sometimes asymmetrical vibrations. The treatment strategy varies according to the onset of the paralysis; for acute cases, conservative management and observation are needed for at least 6 months following the injury; however, this depends on the severity of symptoms, associated dysphagia, and the patient's vocal demands. Other treatment modalities include voice therapy, surgical intervention, and early injection of a temporary material such as hyaluronic acid. Recent studies endorsed early injection as it creates a favorable vocal fold position and reduces the need for laryngeal framework surgeries, in comparison to late injection. Laryngeal framework surgery or vocal fold augmentation with fat or a permanent injection material are indicated for management of permanent or chronic cases [22].

2. *Sulcus vocalis and iatrogenic vocal fold scar:* A condition related to a defect in the surface epithelium of the vocal fold associated with deformity of the lamina propria affecting its pliability, hence causing a stiffness of the mucosa. This defect varies from a superficial invagination to a deep pit with structural deformity of the deep layer of the lamina propria extending to the muscle layer in most cases. Sulcus vocalis is classified into three types: type I involves only an invagination of the surface epithelium extending to the superficial lamina propria; type II (Sulcus Vergeture), the depression, extends to the vocal ligament; type III entails a deep focal pit including the muscle layer. Dysphonia is the main presenting symptom; videolaryngostroboscopy varies from only a faint longitudinal depression on the vocal fold with minimal alteration of the mucosal wave to a deep pit with complete stiffness and atrophy of the mucosa and glottis insufficiency. The treatment plan depends on the type of the sulcus where for symptomatized type 1, vocal fold injection with hyaluronic acid is associated with good results. For type 2, especially cases that are associated with diminished vibration and glottis insufficiency, a submucosal excision of the sulcus is performed through a superficial incision done along the upper margins of the sulcus, and then the edge of the sulcus is gripped by a triangular forceps and proceed with a blunt dissection to free the epithelium from the edge of the sulcus; this is followed by injection medialization of the vocal to counteract glottis insufficiency. In rare occasions, vocal fold vibration is preserved; hence, injection medialization of the vocal fold is sufficient. In type 3, follow the same procedure as in type 2; however, some cases require a graft implantation. Vocal fold scars are a condition where there is deposition of abnormal tissue usually fibrous tissue in the lamina propria with a resultant obliteration of the lamina propria and subsequent atrophy of the vocal fold. Three types are identified; type I involves the lamina propria and the epithelium, type II extends to involve the muscle, whereas type III is characterized by the formation of an anterior glottis web. Vocal fold steroid injection in superficial scars is beneficial as it can stop fibrosis. In type II, it is advisable to do an injection augmentation in addition, whereas type III requires an open subtotal partial laryngectomy [23].

9. Vocal fold injection

It is a procedure that involves placing a substance into the vocal fold to retrieve its vibratory pattern without affecting its morphological and functional characteristics. The indications of vocal fold injection have widened to include superficial injection into the lamina propria for management of vocal fold scars and sulcus vocalis as well as steroid injections for benign vocal fold lesions and deep injection as in vocal fold augmentation or injection medialization laryngoplasty. Vocal fold augmentation aims at the correction of glottis insufficiency whether it is global, as in vocal fold paralysis, paresis, presbyphonia, deep scars, and sulcus vocalis, or focal, as in iatrogenic soft tissue loss [24].

9.1 Injection approaches

There are two major approaches: per-oral and per-cutaneous vocal fold injection approaches.

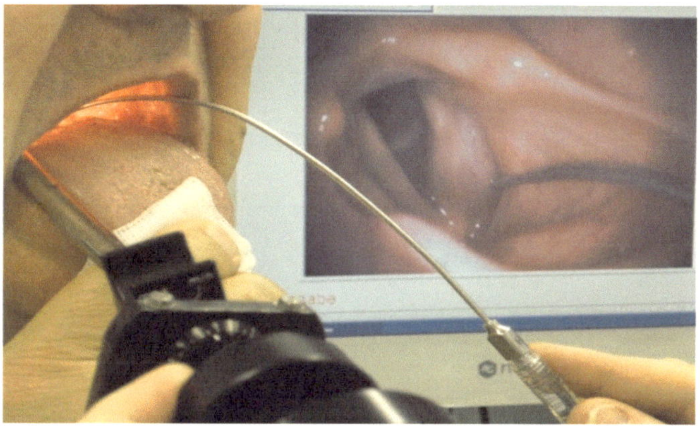

Figure 12.
Per-oral vocal fold injection approach. Physician-assisted visualization by rigid laryngoscope.

1. *Per-oral vocal fold injection approach:* It includes two routes:

2. *Per-oral vocal fold injection under general anesthesia:* Using the traditional suspension microlaryngoscopy: It allows excellent visualization and optimal needle placement. However, it does not provide direct feedback on the amount of the injectable material nor can it assess the patient's voice during the injection [24].

3. *Per-Oral vocal fold injection in the awake setting (Office-based):* This route utilizes a curved laryngeal needle passing from the oral cavity following the curvature of the tongue base through the supraglottis to the vocal fold, thus providing a direct transluminal track into the vocal fold (**Figure 12**).

4. *Visualization:* Either physician-based using a rigid laryngoscope or assistant-based using a flexible laryngoscope.

5. *Anesthesia:*

    - Nasal: Nasal pack is soaked in 4% lidocaine and nasal decongestant to anesthetize the nasal cavity before introducing the flexible laryngoscope.

    - Oropharyngeal: Spraying 10% lidocaine spray onto the lateral and posterior pharyngeal walls.

    - Laryngeal: Through the endoscope side channel, a 3 ml of 4% lidocaine is dropped over the vocal fold while the patient is phonating, which provokes a cough that helps the propagation of the anesthetic agent over the vocal fold and prevents its trans tracheal absorption. If the side-channeled endoscope is not available, an Abraham cannula is used to apply the anesthetic agent. Then using a laryngeal cotton applicator, a cottonoid soaked in 2% lidocaine is used to palpate the vocal fold that is to be injected to ensure that it is well anesthetized (**Figure 13**).

6. *Procedure:* The needle is introduced through the oral cavity and then follows a 90° path into the endolarynx, retracting the ventricular fold laterally to insert the

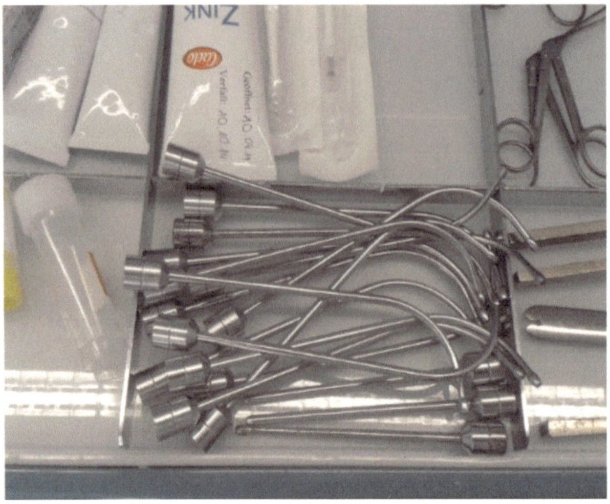

Figure 13.
Abraham curved laryngeal Cannula.

needle into the posterolateral aspect of the vocal fold lateral to the thyroarytenoid muscle. The needle is placed on a depth of 5 mm (to bypass Reinke's space). Care should be taken to avoid deposition of the material in Reinke's space, otherwise it will impede the viscoelastic characteristics of the SLP. The augmentation starts initially on the infraglottic surface and then proceeds to the glottis level (**Figure 14A** and **B** shows the laryngeal needles).

7. *Post-injection care:* The patient is advised to restrict oral intake for at least 1 hour following the injection until the effect of the anesthesia wears off. Complete voice rest is occasionally recommended to avoid extrusion of the material from the injection site.

8. *Advantages and disadvantages:*

    - The technique allows for the precision of the injection site.

    - Suitable for patients with distorted neck anatomy such as large neck scars, thick neck, and cervical spondylosis.

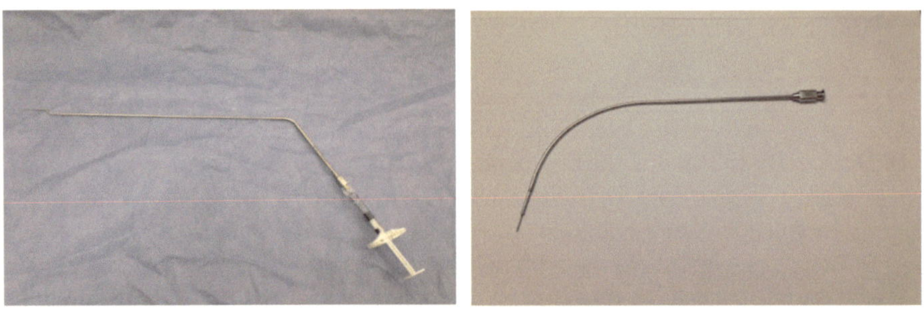

(A) (B)

Figure 14.
Laryngeal needle for per-oral vocal fold injection approach. (A) Under general anesthesia. (B) Under local anesthesia.

- Enables palpation of the cricoarytenoid joint to confirm its fixation.
- It can be used for supraglottic injection as in cases of spasmodic dysphonia.

However,

- The presence of an exaggerated gag reflex may render the procedure potentially difficult.
- The presence of a crowded oropharynx, overhanging arytenoid cartilages, and trismus can prohibit the procedure.
- The procedure may be difficult in patients who are unable to sit still and those with limited limb mobility.

1. Per-cutaneous vocal fold injection approach: The visualization is always assistant-based via a flexible laryngoscope. It includes three routes:

    a. *Trans-Cricothyroid Vocal Fold Injection:* This technique involves the injection through the cricothyroid membrane; it necessitates palpation of the inferior border of the thyroid cartilage. A 25 g needle is inserted 3–7 mm lateral to the midline and directed laterally to reach the vocal folds via the subglottic airway. The skin overlying the cricothyroid may be anesthetized by local infiltration of 1% lidocaine mixed with epinephrine before the procedure.

    b. *Trans-Thyroid Vocal Fold Injection:* A 24 or 25-g needle is introduced through the thyroid cartilage immediately inferior to a point in its middle (3-5 mm lateral to the vocal fold). This technique is suitable for augmentation of the anterior vocal fold; nonetheless, it cannot be done in patients with calcified thyroid cartilage (> 30 years).

    c. *Trans-Thyrohyoid Vocal Fold Injection:* The needle is inserted through the thyrohyoid membrane. A 25 g needle is introduced through the skin overlying the superior thyroid notch and directed downward to enter the larynx at the petiole of the epiglottis. Sometimes, bending the needle at various points renders the procedure easier. (See figure for different needle shapes).

    d. *Upsides and pitfalls:*

        - Per-cutaneous approach is associated with better patient compliance as it is easier to do in patients with exaggerated gag.
        - It is a fast and simple procedure.

However,

- It is a blind approach, especially the trans-cricothyroid injection technique.
- Difficult in obese patients and patients with neck deformities.
- The depth of injection is difficult to be controlled [25].

9.2 Auxiliary vocal fold injection approaches

1. *Trans-Nasal Vocal Fold Injection:* It utilizes a 23–25 gauge flexible needle passing through the working channel of a flexible laryngoscope. This technique is easy to perform and can be used as a substitute for other approaches especially in the presence of patient's limitations. Still, owing to the small diameter of the injection needle, it can accommodate only diluted preparations of the injection materials [26].

2. Other approaches include light-guided injection and ultrasound-guided injection techniques.

3. In conclusion, each vocal fold injection approach requires a certain learning curve, and each surgeon develops his own favorite injection approach; nevertheless, it is beneficial to be oriented with more than one injection technique to be armed against unexpected patient circumstances.

9.3 Injection materials

It is of utmost importance that the material complements the biochemical and viscoelastic properties of the superficial lamina propria. Materials can be classified into three categories:

1. *Temporary materials:*

    - Hyaluronic Acid Derivatives: Can last up to 12 months with some preparations. They are believed to replace the lamina propria in vocal fold scars and sulcus vocalis.

    - Carboxymethylcellulose (Radiesse voice gel): Lasts only 3–4 months [27].

2. *Durable material*

    - Calcium hydroxylapatite: It has a mean duration of 18 months.

    - Polydimethylsiloxane: Vox® Implant. It is biologically safe and a potentially permanent material.

3. *Permanent Materials:*

    - Autologous Fat: Under general anesthesia, fat is prepared through liposuction of at least 60 cc of translucent solution by a liposuction cannula introduced through a 1 cm skin incision in the lower abdomen above the anterior superior iliac spine, and then the solution is centrifuged to separate the fat cells from blood and fatty acids. This procedure should be done under complete aseptic conditions in the operative room. Fat is injected through a high-pressure syringe (Bruening syringe) (**Figure 15**) lateral to the thyroarytenoid muscle or in the paraglottic space. Fat should be over-injected as it is readily absorbed from the injection site [28].

    - Autologous Cartilage: Diced cartilage is injected in the same technique as the autologous fat.

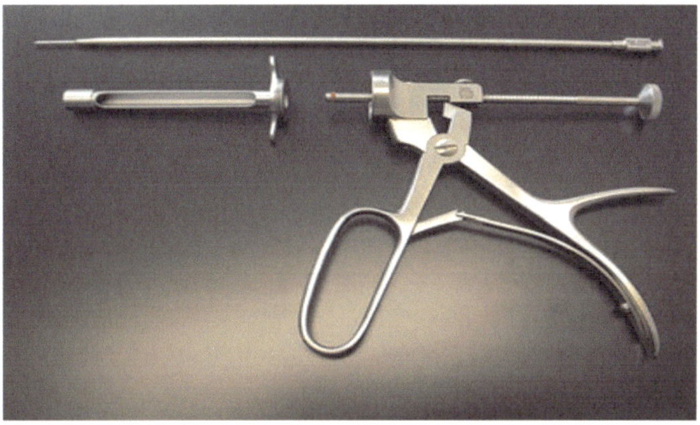

Figure 15.
Fat Injection Bruening syringe.

9.4 Other therapeutic vocal fold injections

1. *Cidofovir and Bevacizumab injection:* These are cytosine nucleotides that inhibit the replication of herpes virus, adenovirus, and human papillomavirus. Cidofovir is injected intralesionally in cases of recurrent respiratory papillomatosis, which is a disease characterized by multiple papillomatous growths involving the larynx and trachea causing dysphonia and airway compromise in severe cases. The disease is of a relapsing nature, and cidofovir is believed to decrease the recurrence rate. The dose is 20–40 mg in less than 4 ml and < 20 mg in less than 2 ml for the pediatric population [29].

2. *Vocal fold steroid injection:* Steroids are powerful inhibitors of inflammation. Local injection of steroids in benign vocal fold lesions has been associated with subsidence of dysphonia as well as reduction of the size of the lesion on videolaryngoscopy. Some surgeons prefer to inject hydrocortisone in the base of the lesion after surgical excision to decrease the risk of occurrence of postoperative scar especially for large-sized lesions with broad bases. Moreover, it can be injected into superficial iatrogenic scars. The value of vocal fold steroid injection is to reduce granulation tissue and hypertrophic scar formation and decrease inflammation. It is best performed via a trans-oral approach under general or local anesthesia. Steroids are injected into the superficial lamina propria, and care must be taken not to extend the injection into the muscle, otherwise a subsequent atrophy may result. Triamcinolone is the preparation to be used mostly (**Figure 16** shows the steps of trans-oral steroid injection for the treatment of bamboo nodes) [30].

9.5 Laryngeal botulinum toxin injection for voice/neurolaryngeal disorders

Botulinum toxin is a neurotoxin produced by *Clostridium botulinum*. When injected into the target muscle, it causes chemical denervation and temporary paralysis by blocking the release of acetylcholine at the motor end plate. Botulinum toxin type A (Botox ® Allergan and Dysport ®) and botulinum toxin type B (Myoblock ®) are the common subtypes available for clinical use, although type A is more durable than type B. The toxin has been used for the management of a variety of voice and

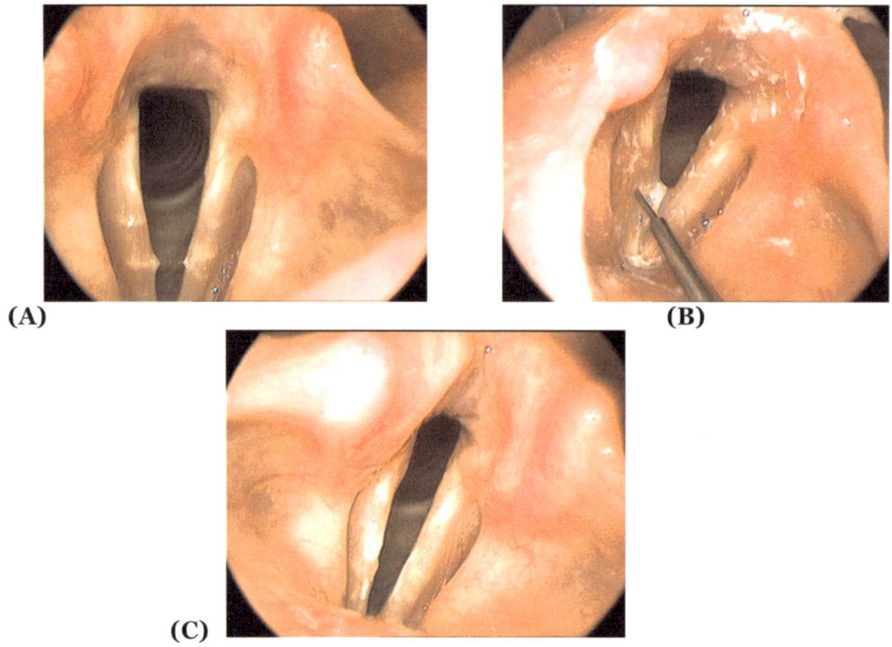

Figure 16.
Videolaryngoscopic view shows per-oral vocal fold injection approach for intralesional steroid injection for bamboo nodes. (A) Shows the pre-injection videolaryngoscopic view, (B) steroid injection in the base of the lesion in the SLP, and (c) one-week post-injection videolaryngoscopic view.

neurolaryngeal disorders such as spasmodic dysphonia, essential voice tremors, paradoxical vocal fold movement, contact granuloma, and bilateral vocal fold immobility. Immediately after botulinum toxin injection, there is a period of severe muscle weakness accompanied by breathy voice and occasional dysphagia persisting for several days, which is then followed by a stable phase of the desired level of muscle weakness lasting from 3 to 4 months.

9.6 Spasmodic dysphonia

Focal laryngeal dystonia has three distinct types: adductor spasmodic dysphonia (ADSD), which is characterized by inappropriate glottis closure resulting in a strained strangled voice; abductor spasmodic dysphonia (ABSD), where there is improper glottis opening leading to breathy voice and hypophonia; and combined adductor and abductor spasmodic dysphonia. Botulinum toxin injection is the treatment of choice where it is injected into the thyroarytenoid/lateral cricoarytenoid muscle complex in ADSD, while it is injected into the posterior cricoarytenoid muscle in ABSD. It can be injected via the per-oral or per-cutaneous approaches under videolaryngoscopic visualization or through an EMG-guided per-cutaneous approach with monitoring of the motor unit action potential. The dose depends on the severity of symptoms; however, an initial dose of 2.5 IU/0.1 ml saline is recommended. The combined glottic and supraglottic injection is preferable as it decreases the breathy voice quality that may accompany the toxin injection and preserves the singing voice pitch in many patients. Subsequent doses are determined according to the clinical response, duration, and frequency of post-injection complications. Other treatment modalities include thyroarytenoid muscle myoneurectomy, type II thyroplasty, and recurrent laryngeal nerve transection; however, these procedures are not within the scope of this chapter [31].

9.7 Essential voice tremors

Rhythmic involuntary movement of the vocal fold during phonation that occurs in isolation or in conjunction with spasmodic dysphonia. Characterized by pitch breaks and vocal arrests or in severe forms, patients may adopt a whispering mode of phonation. Botulinum toxin can be injected into the TA muscle with a dose of 3.7 IU in each side to decrease the amplitude of tremors [32].

9.8 Paradoxical vocal fold movement

Paroxysmal periods of adduction of the vocal fold during inspiration leading to episodic inspiratory stridor. Several factors are involved in the etiology including GERD, brain stem compression or conversion disorders, and allergic rhinitis. Treatment includes alleviating coexisting conditions such as treatment of GERD and nasal allergy, breathing exercises, and botulinum toxin injection dosing of 10 IU in each vocal fold in severe refractory cases [33].

9.9 Bilateral vocal fold immobility

It is a serious life-threatening condition that results from bilateral injury of the recurrent laryngeal nerve that may be caused by anterior neck surgery, commonly thyroidectomy, and less common causes such as neurogenic diseases and infectious etiology. Stridor is the most common presentation and less frequently dysphonia and dysphagia. Patients traditionally undergo tracheostomy to improve ventilation and alleviate stridor. After RLN injury, there is a tendency to misdirect reinnervation of the adductor muscles by inspiratory fibers, and this reinnervation causes hyperadduction of the vocal fold and a resultant stridor. Botulinum toxin injection into the TA/LCA muscle complex weakens the force of adductory muscles and laryngeal closure, allowing an increased patency of the airway and rebalancing the position of the paralyzed vocal folds by using the unopposed pull of the abductor muscles into a more abducted position. Each vocal fold is injected by 5 IU of BTX, yielding a static airway widening. Alternative treatment options include cordotomy, arytenoidectomy, suture lateralization of the vocal fold, and type II thyroplasty; however, they are associated with dysphonia in many cases. On the other hand, botulinum toxin injection creates a balance between preserving voice and maintaining an adequate airway. Nevertheless, it is a temporary procedure, and patients may need repeated injections [34].

10. Endoscopic laser-assisted surgery of the vocal fold

Laser stands for "light amplification by stimulated emission of radiation." There are a variety of lasers used in the treatment of head and neck pathologies that differ in their wave lengths; however, CO_2 laser is the most widely used type in laryngeal pathologies. Carbon dioxide laser produces continuous or pulsed waves, which can be used to dissect the tissues like a scalpel or to evaporate lesions. It can be used in cases of benign or malignant lesions of the vocal fold, glottis or subglottic stenosis, vascular lesions of the vocal fold, recurrent respiratory papillomatosis, and arytenoidectomy or transverse cordectomy in treatment of bilateral vocal fold paralysis. Its advantages include minimal intraoperative bleeding and better hemostasis, less tissue damage, and less manipulation of tissues than the cold surgical dissection; nonetheless, the prerequisite for the successful laser procedure is consistent adherence to the safety protocol. This safety protocol includes operative room safety comprising moistened eye pads for patients, laser-protected ETT, saline-filled ETT balloon for airway protection, and protection of the OR personnel through the use of protection eye glasses. It also includes insuring the safety of the adjacent tissues against collateral heat damage by applying moist cottonoid pads. In addition, a suction tube is used to absorb the vaporized smoke to maintain a clean surgical field [35, 36].

10.1 Laser microlaryngoscopy for benign lesions of the vocal fold

Can be performed via a trans-oral approach under general anesthesia or in the awake settings through a flexible endoscope with a working side-channel. Using the same surgical technique mentioned in the cold microsurgical instrumentation with an additional saline-soaked cottonoid placed in the subglottic region, the lesion is grasped with microforceps, and CO_2 laser is used to ablate the lesion on a superficial plane. Caution should be applied to avoid damage of the deeper structure of the mucosa or muscle layers. Topical lidocaine is applied onto the vocal fold to avoid post-intubation laryngospasm, and systemic steroids are advised to reduce the possible inflammation following the surgery [37].

10.2 Recurrent respiratory papillomatosis

Utilizing the traditional suspension microlaryngoscopy, the laser beam is used to evaporate the lesion superficially. A suction tube is used to remove the excess charred material emitted from the laser evaporation [38].

10.3 Vocal fold vascular lesions

Carbon dioxide laser is used to cauterize the dilated blood vessels. If the lesion is located on the vibratory area of the vocal fold, the laser beam should be directed tangentially to the free edges [36].

10.4 Anterior Glottic web

Under visualization of the suspension microlaryngoscopy and enhanced by a 30° or 70° telescope, CO_2 laser is used to divide the web to approximately 1 mm deep into the interior surface of the thyroid cartilage. This is followed by the application of a keel to prevent the re-adhesion of the web; the keel is tailored according to the distance between the superior and inferior extension of the web and is fixed to the anterior neck by a prolene suture using the Lichtenberger endo-extralaryngeal needle passer. The keel is removed 10–14 days later after ensuring a complete healing of the mucosa [36].

1. Other applications such as lesions affecting the airway including posterior glottis stenosis, cordectomy or arytenoidectomy in bilateral vocal fold paralysis are beyond the scope of this chapter that is dedicated to lesions of the vocal folds affecting the voice.

2. Laser is one of the resources used in vocal fold endoscopic surgeries; it is falsely believed that it is better than cold surgical instruments with regards to the accuracy and distinctness of the procedure; on the contrary, it carries the risk of collateral heat damage that may be associated with its use [39].

Author details

Reham Abdel Wakil Ibrahim
Department of Otorhinolaryngology, Unit of Phoniatrics, Assiut University Faculty of Medicine, El Fateh, Assiut, Egypt

*Address all correspondence to: dr.reham.ibrahim@gmail.com

References

[1] Fried M, Meller S. Adult Laryngeal Anatomy: The Larynx (edited by Marvin F). St Louis: Mosby-Year Book Inc; 1996. pp. 25-32

[2] Hirano M. Structure and vibratory behavior of the vocal fold. In: Sawashima M, Cooper F, editors. Dynamic Aspects of Speech Production. Tokyo, Japan: University of Tokyo; 1977. pp. 13-30

[3] Bryant NJ et al. Human posterior cricoarytenoid muscle compartments: Anatomy and mechanics. Archives of Otolaryngology. 1996;**122**:1331

[4] Estill J, Mcdonald MK, Obert K, Steinhauer KM. Level two workbook. Figure combination for six voice qualities, 2nd ed. Estill Voice International. Pittsburgh: Pennsylvania Incorporated Company; 2019

[5] Hirano M, Kakita Y. Cover-body theory of vocal fold vibration. In: Speech Science. San Diego: College-Hill Press; 1985

[6] Hirano M. Clinical Examination of the Voice. Berlin, Heidelberg, New York: Springer; 1981

[7] Dejonckere PH, Crevier L, Elbaz E, et al. Clinical implementation of a multidimensional basic protocol for assessing functional results of voice therapy. In: Jahnke K, Fischer M, editors. Proceedings of the 4th EUFOS Congress; Berlin. 2000. pp. 561-565

[8] Angerstein W, Baracca G, Dejonckere Ph, Echternach M, et al. Diagnosis and differential diagnosis of voice disorders. In: Zehnhoff-Dinnesen AA, et al., editors. Phoniatrics I, European Manual of Medicine. Berlin, Heidelberg, Dordrecht, and New York city: Springer; 2020. pp. 349-430

[9] Karnell MP, Melton SD, Childers JM, et al. Reliability of clinician-based (GRBAS and CAPE-V) and patient-based (V-RQOL and IPVI) documentation of voice disorders. Journal of Voice. 2007;**21**(5):576-590.32

[10] Dejonckere PH, Bradley P, Clemente P, Cornut G, et al. A basic protocol for functional assessment of voice pathology especially for investigating the efficacy of (Phonosurgical) treatments and evaluating new assessment techniques. Guidelines elaborated by the committee of Phoniatrics of the European laryngological society (ELS). European Archives of Oto-Rhino-Laryngology. 2001;**258**:77-82

[11] Wendler J, Rauhut A, Krüger H. Classification of voice qualities**Dedicated to Prof. Dr. Med. Peter Biesalski on the occasion of his 70th birthday. Journal of Phonetics. 1986;**14**(3):483-488. DOI: 10.1016/S0095-4470(19)30694-1

[12] Béquignon E, Bach C, Fugain C, Guilleré L, et al. Long term results of surgical treatment of vocal fold nodules. The Laryngoscope. 2013;**123**(8):1926-1930

[13] Verdolini K, Rosen CA, Branski R. Classification Manual of Voice Disorders. Mahwah, NJ: Lawrence Erlbaum Associates; 2005

[14] Bouchayer M, Cornut G. Microsurgical treatment of benign vocal fold lesions: Indications, technique, results. Folia Phoiniatr. 1992;**44**:155-184

[15] Courey MS, Gardner GM, Stone RE, Ossoff RH. Endoscopic vocal fold microflap: A three-year experience. The

Annals of Otology, Rhinology, and Laryngology. 1995;**104**(Pt. 1):267-273

[16] Zeitels SM, Hillman RE, Bunting GW, Vaughn T. Reinke's edema: Phonatory mechanisms and management strategies. The Annals of Otology, Rhinology, and Laryngology. 1997;**106**:533-543

[17] Gökcan KM, Dursun G. Vascular lesions of the vocal fold. European Archives of Oto-Rhino-Laryngology. 2009;**266**:527-533

[18] Zeitels SM. Premalignant epithelium and microinvasive cancer of the vocal fold: The evolution of phonomicrosurgical management. Laryngoscope. 1995;**105**:1-51

[19] Simpson CB, Hoffman MR. Principles of phonosurgery. International Journal of Head and Neck Surgery. 2021;**12**(4):144-152

[20] Sharma S, Patel R, Hasmi MF, Friede R. (2023): 3-3-2 Rule. In: StatPearls [Internet]. Treasure Island (FL): StatPearls Publishing; 2024. 2023 Aug 17. PMID: 29630287. Book Shelf: NBK493235

[21] Al Yaghchi C, Onwordi LN. Airway glottis insufficiency. In: StatPearls [Internet]. Treasure Island (FL): StatPearls Publishing; 2023, 2024

[22] Kupfer RA, Meyer TK. Evaluation of unilateral vocal fold immobility. Current Otorhinolaryngology Reports. 2014;**2**: 105-113

[23] Miaśkiewicz B, Szkiełkowska A, Gos E, Panasiewicz A, et al. Pathological sulcus vocalis: Treatment approach and voice outcomes in 36 patients. European Archives of Oto-Rhino-Laryngology. 2018;**275**:2763-2771

[24] Mallur PS, Rosen CA. Vocal fold injection: Review of indications, techniques, and materials for augmentation. Clinical and Experimental Otorhinolaryngology. 2010;**3**(4):177-182

[25] Anderson TD, Mirza N. Immediate percutaneous medialization for acute vocal fold immobility with aspiration. The Laryngoscope. 2001;**111**:1318-1321

[26] Trask DK, Shellenberger DL, Hoffman HT. Transnasal, endoscopic vocal fold augmentation. The Laryngoscope. 2005;**115**:2262-2265

[27] Mallur PS, Morrison MP, Postma GN, Amin MR, Rosen CA. Safety and efficacy of carboxymethylcellulose in the treatment of glottis insufficiency. The Laryngoscope. 2012;**122**(2):322-326

[28] Truzzi GM, Pauna HF, Bette P, Gusmão RJ, et al. Methods of fat tissue processing for human vocal fold injection: A systematic review. Journal of Voice. 2017;**31**(2):244.e17-244.e21

[29] Snoeck R, Wellens W, Desloovere C, et al. Treatment of severe laryngeal papillomatosis with intralesional injections of cidofovir [(S)-1-(3-hydroxy-2-phosphonylmethoxypropyl) cytosine]. Journal of Medical Virology. 1998;**54**(3):219-225

[30] Campagnolo AM, Tsuji HD, Sennes LU, Imamura R. Steroid injection in chronic inflammatory vocal fold disorders, literature review. Revista Brasileira de Otorrinolaringologia. 2008; **74**(6):926-932

[31] Blitzer A. Spasmodic dysphonia and botulinum toxin: Experience from the largest treatment series. European Journal of Neurology. 2010;**17**(Suppl. 1): 28-30. DOI: 10.1111/j.1468-1331.2010.03047.x

[32] Sullivan KL, Hauser RA, Zesiewicz TA. Essential tremor: Epidemiology,

diagnosis, and treatment. The Neurologist. 2003;**10**:250-258

[33] Maschka D, Bauman NM, McCray PB, et al. A classification scheme for paradoxical vocal cord motion. Laryngoscope. 1997;**107**:1429-1435

[34] Ibrahim RAE, Aboshanif M, Farghaly S. Botulinum toxin injection in bilateral vocal fold immobility. Egyptian Journal of Neck Surgery and Otorhinolaryngology. 2020;**6**(2):11-19

[35] Buckmire R et al. Lasers in laryngology. In: Merati AL, Bielamowicz SA, editors. Textbook of Laryngology. San Diego: Plural; 2006. pp. 190-199

[36] Yan Y, Olszewski A, Hoffman M, Zhuang P, Ford C, Dailey S, et al. Use of lasers in laryngeal surgery. Journal of Voice. 2010;**24**(1):102-109

[37] Benninger MS. Microdissection or microspot CO_2 laser for limited vocal fold benign lesions: A prospective randomized trial. Laryngoscope. 2000; **110**:1-17

[38] Zeitels S, Anderson R, et al. Office-based 532-nm pulsed KTP laser treatment of glottal papillomatosis and dysplasia. The Annals of Otology, Rhinology, and Laryngology. 2006;**115**: 679-685

[39] Milczuk HA, Smith JD, Everts EC. Congenital laryngeal webs: Surgical management and clinical embryology. International Journal of Pediatric Otorhinolaryngology. 2000;**52**:1-9

Chapter 2

Ground-Level Alternobaric Vertigo: A Contemporary Perspective on Eustachian Tube Dysfunction and Balance

Hee-Young Kim

Abstract

This chapter delves into Ground-Level Alternobaric Vertigo (GLAV), with a particular emphasis on its interaction with Eustachian Tube Dysfunction (ETD). GLAV's prevalence under normal ground-level conditions is gaining attention, highlighting the need for improved understanding and clinical differentiation. Our investigation begins with an examination of GLAV etiology and symptoms before moving on to the evolution of diagnostic and treatment techniques. We track the route from first misdiagnoses to improved comprehension, using sophisticated diagnostics such as tympanometry and encouraging Eustachian tube catheterization. The incorporation of current breakthroughs in GLAV detection and therapy is an important component of this chapter. This includes a full assessment of innovative pharmacological therapies and tactics for managing middle ear cavity pressure, emphasizing the necessity of continuous research for increased diagnostic precision and knowledge of long-term effects. The chapter's contribution is to advocate for a reevaluation of historical and contemporary vertigo cases for correct diagnosis. It promotes the use of tympanometry in diagnostic protocols and emphasizes the need of joint research in the field of vestibular diseases. This all-encompassing approach makes the chapter an essential resource for healthcare practitioners and academics, matching the dynamic growth of medical knowledge and practices in vestibular sciences.

Keywords: ground-level alternobaric vertigo, Eustachian tube dysfunction, vestibular disorders, middle ear pressure, tympanometry, Eustachian tube catheterization, vestibular function test, laryngopharyngeal reflux

1. Introduction

1.1 Opening statement

At the core of our discourse on ground-level alternobaric vertigo (GLAV) rests a compelling paradox: a condition that is critical to our comprehension of vestibular disorders (VD) yet often escapes notice in everyday clinical practice (**Figure 1**).

This dichotomy is not merely a gap in scholarly discussion; it is a fundamental deficiency in addressing patient health concerns.

The clinical manifestation of GLAV is obscure, and its symptoms may be erroneously ascribed to more frequently diagnosed conditions such as Meniere's disease, benign paroxysmal positional vertigo (BPPV) or otolithiasis, vestibular neuritis, vestibular migraine, vertebrogenic dizziness, persistent postural-perceptual dizziness (PPPD), as well as central disorders, and others, if a high level of suspicion is not utilized. This event leads to its frequent misclassification as idiopathic vertigo, highlighting a significant oversight in current diagnostic approaches.

This chapter endeavors to bring GLAV into the spotlight, emphasizing its rightful recognition in the differential diagnosis of VD. Originating from mild Eustachian tube dysfunction (ETD), GLAV presents a diagnostic conundrum. Its proper understanding is essential, not just for academic rigor but, more importantly, for its profound implications in patient care. The unpredictable nature of GLAV symptoms can disrupt daily life activities, leading to a decline in the overall quality of life. A precise diagnosis, therefore, is pivotal for effective treatment strategies, avoiding the pitfalls of misdiagnosis and suboptimal management.

Our goal is to unravel the complexities surrounding GLAV. We aim to shift the clinical focus toward this often-misunderstood condition, enhancing the quality of care for patients grappling with this challenging VD.

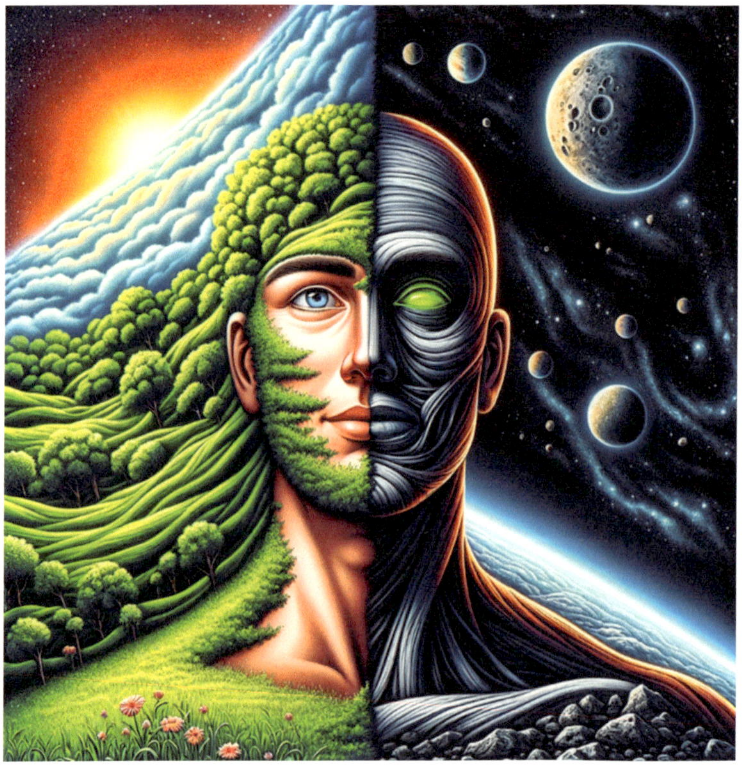

Figure 1.
A Surreal Depiction of Ground-Level Alternobaric Vertigo (GLAV) – This illustration metaphorically represents the dichotomy of GLAV as experienced on Earth versus a distorted gravitational perception akin to another planet. It visually conveys the paradox of a critical yet often clinically overlooked vestibular condition, embodying the dual sensory experiences that define GLAV.

1.2 Definition of GLAV

In the realm of VD, GLAV stands out as a unique and often misunderstood entity. It appears as a distinct clinical condition characterized by asymmetric vestibular function due to unequal middle ear pressures (MEP) at ground level [1]. Alternobaric vertigo (ABV) can occur when a pilot's or diver's passive opening MEP during an ascent or descent is not the same in both ears at the same height [2]. GLAV often results from minor atmospheric pressure fluctuations worsened by ETD, and it is characterized by vertigo or dizziness that does not involve the dramatic pressure or altitude changes seen in the conventional ABV [3]. GLAV's hallmark is its occurrence at ground level, highlighting its sensitivity to even small variances in MEP. This condition can significantly disrupt balance and orientation, affecting daily life and underscoring the labyrinthine mechanism's sensitivity in the inner ear. Understanding GLAV's unique characteristics is crucial for correct diagnosis and effective management in the realm of VD.

1.3 Brief overview of GLAV

GLAV presents a clinical conundrum, challenging traditional feelings of VD and shedding light on the complex relationship between ET function and vestibular balance. This condition, characterized by vertigo due to subtle variations in MEP, underlines the importance of ET in keeping vestibular equilibrium. GLAV's sporadic symptoms, often triggered during routine activities, need a nuanced understanding among clinicians for a correct diagnosis and tailored treatment strategies. Recognizing and addressing GLAV in clinical practice can significantly improve the quality of life for those affected, offering relief from the disorder's disorienting and unsettling impacts.

2. Historical context

2.1 Discussion on Nicolas Deleau's 1837 report and its implications

The foundation of our historical understanding of GLAV is profoundly anchored in the pioneering work of Nicolas Deleau in 1837 [4]. Deleau's report, originally perceived in the context of Meniere's disease [5], is now acknowledged as arguably the earliest clinical description that correlates with what we now know as GLAV. Deleau's observations were groundbreaking at the time. He described a clinical picture that included dizziness, tinnitus, hearing impairment, a feeling of pressure in the ear, disordered movements of the eyeballs, eye pain, deteriorating vision, and vomiting, which he treated with ETC and an air douche—a technique that improved the symptoms.

Deleau described the experience of Philippine Philippe, a thirty-seven-year-old cook, in one of his cases. She suffered from persistent symptoms such as eye pain from childhood until the age of fourteen, as well as ringing in the ears and eventual deafness, particularly in the left ear, a few years after her menstrual periods began. Her acute symptoms included dizziness, which was unsuccessfully treated with cautery to the arm, and episodes of dizziness followed by vomiting between the ages of twenty-four and twenty-six. Despite general and local bloodletting helped by purgatives, these episodes persisted until June 28, 1836. Deleau's treatment, which included tube catheterization and air douche over two days, reduced her dizziness and improved her hearing and sight.

This method was pioneering, implying a clear link between ETD and vertiginous symptoms, a concept that was not widely acknowledged or understood at the time [4, 5]. The importance of Deleau's study resides in its unintended revelation of GLAV decades before the name or idea was publicly recognized. His study alluded to the relevance of the ET in sustaining not only auditory function but also balance. This early link between ETD and vertigo calls into question the later, more narrow focus on the vestibular system alone in explaining vertiginous symptoms.

Incorrectly reading Deleau's observations as Meniere's disease rather than GLAV reflects the historical pattern of misunderstanding and undervaluing the importance of GLAV in vertigo, particularly in practical contexts. This occurrence exemplifies a broader tendency in the field of medical history, in which innovative understandings frequently remain hidden in incorrectly understood data, awaiting reevaluation and right categorization. Deleau's observations have substantial ramifications in modern therapeutic practice. They serve as a reminder of the complexities of vertigo and VD and the importance of recognizing ETD as a main factor in the differential diagnosis of vertigo. His report recommends for a more holistic approach to detecting and treating vertigo, one that acknowledges the ET's function in vestibular health. Deleau's work thus not only contributes to the historical narrative of GLAV but also conveys important lessons for modern medicine: the need of holistic assessment in VD and the possibility for historical medical reports to inform and enhance present understanding and practice.

2.2 Evolution of understanding in the field

A rich history of understanding and scientific advancements surrounds GLAV and its relationship with ETD. This subsection explores the journey from early recognition to contemporary perspectives, highlighting how our comprehension of GLAV and ETD has transformed over the years.

2.2.1 Early observations and theories

There has been a gradual and significant evolution of understanding on the road to understanding GLAV in the fields of otolaryngology and vestibular medicine. Since the early observations of Nicolas Deleau in 1837, our comprehension of GLAV and its relationship with ETD has undergone a transformative journey, shaping the modern approach to VD. In the years following Deleau's report, the focus in vestibular medicine was primarily on the inner ear mechanisms, with a limited appreciation for the role of the ET. Common VDs such as Meniere disease and BPPV dominated clinical attention, while the subtleties of GLAV remained largely unrecognized.

2.2.2 Adam Politzer's contribution to ETC

A significant figure in the mid-nineteenth-century otology, Adam Politzer, performed critical studies on the ear's nerve supply and the pressure effects of the tympanic cavity on the labyrinth in 1861 [6]. Simultaneously, he conducted extensive microscopic inspections of the labyrinth, fostering professional relationships that advanced otological knowledge. These investigations contributed to a better understanding of auditory mechanics and balance. Politzer's ideas extended beyond theoretical studies to practical applications, most notably his invention of the eponymous

Politzerization in 1863. This method was designed to ensure the functionality of the ET, providing a less invasive alternative to the then-common ETC. Politzer's method permitted non-invasive middle ear inflation by injecting a puff of air into the patient's nostril while swallowing, simplifying the process of balancing middle ear and nasopharyngeal pressures, and furthering the treatment of ETD [7].

Politzer's passion for improving ETC procedures was clear throughout his tenure. His ongoing clinical trials and collaborations, particularly with Josef Gruber, have significantly advanced the treatment of ETD. Despite Gruber's proposal of the term "Valsalva's passive experiment" in 1870 as an alternative to "Politzer's method," which Gruber did not favor, Politzer's techniques eventually gained wider recognition. Gruber's contributions, while valuable, notably his version of the insufflation airbag, did not achieve the long-term reputation that Politzer's methods earned [8]. To summarize, Adam Politzer's contributions to ETC were critical in defining the present approach to vestibular medicine. His study not only gave a deeper understanding of the physiology of the ear, but it also revolutionized the practical treatment of diseases connected to the ET, creating a new standard in the field.

2.2.3 James Yearsley's perspective on systemic influences on ear health

James Yearsley's work "Deafness Practically Illustrated," published in 1863, introduced the new concept of "stomach deafness," in which he linked gastrointestinal issues to the functioning of the ET [9]. Yearsley postulated that disorders such as gastroesophageal reflux (GERD), laryngopharyngeal reflux (LPR), and nasopharyngeal reflux (NPR) could have a major impact on auditory health. Recent research has backed up this theory by finding a relationship between systemic health and otolaryngological problems. His understanding of the multifaceted character of ETD includes what is now recognized as reflux-related inflammation, broadening the etiological spectrum of ear disorders [9].

2.2.4 Peter Allen's progressive insights and the onset of modern otolaryngology

Peter Allen is remembered in the history of otolaryngology for his fundamental work in 1871, which represented a critical turn toward contemporary study in the profession. Allen provided unique insights into the specific situation of VD, building on the fundamental work of forefathers such as Adam Politzer, who established the impact of tympanic cavity pressure on the labyrinth. His talks, particularly on "Aural Catarrh," shed light on the complexity of ETD and its profound consequences for vertigo. Allen's work into the intricacies of intra-auricular pressure—notably its impact on labyrinth fluid—was a game changer, showing the direct influence of these pressure changes on vestibular symptoms. This trailblazing viewpoint was crucial in creating modern knowledge of VD, establishing such pressure fluctuations as a cornerstone notion in current otolaryngological practice [10].

Allen bridged the gap between the historical insights supplied by a pioneer like James Yearsley and the then-nascent modern techniques by focusing on the significance of intratympanic and intralabyrinthine pressures in the field of vertigo. His contributions were more than incremental; they were a quantum leap in the science of otolaryngology, foreshadowing principles that remain basic in the assessment and treatment of ear-related balance problems. In this sense, Peter Allen's legacy goes beyond that of a historical figure. He is regarded as a visionary whose intellectual daring created the groundwork for future otological inquiry and invention. Many sophisticated practices that are important to modern otolaryngological care were foreshadowed by his thoughts on the inner workings of the ear, particularly the importance of ET in vestibular health. Allen's commitment to increasing medical understanding and practice has been critical in setting the way for a richer, more educated engagement with vestibular health issues [10].

2.3 Twentieth century: a focus on ET obstruction

The twentieth century witnessed a growing interest in the complexities of the vestibular system, with advancements in diagnostic technologies and a deeper understanding of vestibular pathophysiology. However, the connection between ETD and vertigo, particularly at ground level, remained underexplored. GLAV, with its elusive and often non-specific symptoms, continued to be overshadowed by more prominent vestibular conditions.

In 1942, F.W. Merica supplied more elucidation by characterizing vertigo as a manifestation of ET obstruction during the mid-twentieth century. This distinction marked a significant moment, linking historical data with a rising awareness of how dysregulated MEP could lead to VD, thus laying the groundwork for the contemporary diagnosis of GLAV [11].

The trajectory of the GLAV story underwent a notable shift following the introduction of the term "alternobaric vertigo" by Dr. Claes Lundgren in 1965. Lundgren's research initially focused on the manifestation of symptoms in divers and aviators resulting from significant fluctuations in barometric pressure [3, 12]. In the historical exploration of VD, particularly ABV, a significant development is the understanding of its occurrence in pilots. ABV in pilots is a specific manifestation of VD that arises from unequal MEP during ascent. Notably, ABV can occur when a pilot's passive opening of MEP is not symmetrical in both ears at the same altitude [2, 12]. This phenomenon has been pivotal in shaping our understanding of ABV, as it highlights the crucial role of ET function in keeping vestibular balance, especially under changing atmospheric conditions. This understanding has not only advanced the field of otolaryngology but also has significant implications for the safety and well-being of pilots and other individuals exposed to similar conditions. This work set up a precedent for finding comparable vestibular reactions arising from the less pronounced pressure changes met at ground level.

It was not until the late twentieth and early twenty-first centuries that a more holistic view began to emerge, integrating the role of the ET in the diagnosis and treatment of vertigo. This shift was driven by a combination of factors: an increase in clinical research, improved diagnostic techniques like the several kinds of vestibular function tests (VFT), and a growing recognition of the limitations of existing approaches to addressing all forms of vertigo.

2.4 The modern era: the emergence of GLAV

The contemporary knowledge of GLAV owes largely to Dr. Bluestone's seminal study. His research revealed the chronic Toynbee phenomenon, which causes persistent swallowing while suffering from nasal congestion, and its link to GLAV. Notably, his research shed light on the treatment of ETD and accompanying symptoms, implying the possible benefits of ETC.

Several major discoveries emerged from Dr. Bluestone's research:

The relationship between persistent ABV at ground level and abnormal VFT results.

It has been established that restoring bilateral MEP can improve vestibular function and alleviate vertigo symptoms.

The realization is that tympanostomy tubes do not always restore normal ET function.

Dr. Bluestone's demand for comprehensive ET function testing emphasized the fact that ETD is a spectrum condition with a wide range of causes and manifestations. His efforts have advanced our understanding of GLAV and affected the larger approach to ETD treatment, emphasizing the relevance of ET function in the diagnosis and management of vestibular disorders [1].

2.5 Looking back and moving forward: advances in research and treatment

In the evolving narrative of GLAV, a crucial turning point has been the reevaluation of historical cases, including Deleau's report. This reexamination, primarily driven by a few researchers, including myself, has brought new insights into the significance of ETD in vertigo. This shift in perspective has contributed to a more sophisticated understanding of GLAV, positioning it not merely as a VD but as a condition significantly influenced by the functionality of the ET. An appreciation for the intricate interaction between the ET and the vestibular system today marks the understanding of GLAV. This recognition has paved the way for more comprehensive diagnostic approaches and targeted treatment strategies, moving beyond the conventional focus on the inner ear alone.

The evolution of understanding in the field of VD, particularly regarding GLAV, illustrates the dynamic nature of medical knowledge. It highlights the importance of continual reevaluation and integration of historical insights with contemporary research, ensuring a holistic and informed approach to patient care. The existing comprehension of GLAV is built upon a diverse range of intellectual curiosity and scientific investigation. Each of these researchers, from Deleau to Bluestone, offered crucial insights, effectively bridging centuries of medical thought, and defining a trajectory that has revolutionized the approach to ETD and balance problems. Their legacies live on in every modern treatment protocol for GLAV, a lasting tribute to the enduring force of medical development.

3. Etiology and pathophysiology

Understanding the etiology and pathophysiology of VD, particularly those related to ETD, is essential for correct diagnosis and effective treatment. This section incorporates key insights from notable studies, supplying a comprehensive overview. Evaluating the ET's functionality is the first essential step in realizing that ETD is a complex spectrum of disorders. It is not just about the tube being overly tight or excessively open. This spectrum includes a variety of conditions, each with its own distinct causes and implications for health [13]. Alernobaric Vertigo (ABV), a VD associated with ETD in pilots or divers, often occurs because of unsynchronized MEP opening in both ears during ascent, resulting in symptoms such as vertigo [12]. Tjernström's study underlines the significance of pilots maintaining balanced MEP [2].

3.1 Mechanisms leading to ETD

ETD is caused by a mix of variables and triggers and can range in severity from little disorientation to intense, devastating episodes. Among the mechanisms that contribute to ETD are:

Certain anatomical variations can interfere with ET function. Among these are nasopharyngeal carcinoma, a cancer of the upper throat, and tumors of the middle cranial fossa. Conditions such as infections or allergies can cause transient or chronic ETD. GERD, LPR, and NPR can all produce inflammation and contribute to ETD. Sudden variations in air pressure, such as those experienced during flights, diving, elevating, or weather events, might put the ET's ability to control MEP to the test, potentially resulting in GLAV. Variations in barometric pressure can worsen ETD even at ground level. Factors such as allergic reactions, sinus infections, and common colds can cause inflammation and congestion, restricting ET function. Furthermore, habits such as sniffing, heavy lifting, formidable Valsalva maneuvers, or drinking water before lying down can aggravate ETD and cause GLAV episodes [14–16].

It is critical to distinguish between "Eustachian tube dysfunction" and "Eustachian tube obstruction." While obstruction refers to physical blockages, ETD comprises a broader range of both obstructive and functional problems. Understanding this distinction is crucial for guiding suitable treatment techniques and grasping the full range of ET-related disorders [16].

3.2 Impact on middle ear and vestibular system

ETD leads to imbalances in MEP, affecting the vestibular and auditory systems. This can result in dizziness, balance issues, and auditory disturbances. Both positive and negative pressure scenarios, akin to ascending or descending in altitude, disrupt hearing and balance mechanics. In cases of GLAV, the ETD-induced pressure imbalance in the middle ear causes abnormal stimulation of the vestibular system. The unequal pressures on either side of the tympanic membrane can create a distorted transmission of sound waves, leading to the vestibular symptoms of GLAV, such as dizziness and balance issues [1, 12, 17, 18].

3.2.1 Positive MEP state at ground level (similar to ascending state)

When the ET becomes obstructed in cases of positive MEP, like that experienced by divers or aviators, a unique challenge arises. Because there is insufficient positive pressure in the middle ear to force the tube open, this obstruction prevents the equalization of even minor positive pressures within the middle ear. Mechanical and hydraulic disturbances in the cochlea and vestibular organs can result from the resulting imbalance. The strain on the tympanic membrane and ossicular chain caused by this unabated positive pressure can impair sound transmission and cause dysregulation and symptoms like aural fullness, tinnitus, and hearing loss. This condition can mimic barotrauma and aggravate GLAV symptoms, especially if the ET still is obstructed, preventing pressure relief [12, 17, 18].

3.2.2 Negative MEP at ground level (similar to descending state)

Negative MEP, typically experienced during descent, can manifest at ground level due to ETD. This leads to a failure to equalize the increasing ambient pressure, creating a vacuum effect in the middle ear. The inward retraction of the tympanic membrane disrupts the ossicular chain and inner ear window dynamics. This results in abnormal fluid movements within the labyrinth, causing the disorienting symptoms of vertigo and the imbalance characteristic of GLAV [12, 17, 18].

3.3 Pathophysiological outcomes and long-term effects of ETD

The major effect of ETD is a disruption in pressure regulation in the middle ear, which results in vestibular disturbances such as vertigo. This dysfunction can progress to middle ear barotrauma and harm the vestibular nerve, resulting in impaired balance and spatial orientation. Chronic ETD may result in fluid buildup in the middle ear, exacerbating vestibular symptoms.

Long-term symptoms of GLAV because of ETD include persistent vertigo, dizziness, and gastrointestinal disease which can considerably affect everyday activities [1, 11]. Prolonged pressure imbalances can cause hearing loss and tinnitus. The persistence of these symptoms can cause psychological stress, such as anxiety and depression, as well as cognitive challenges such as concentration and recall issues [1, 19]. Balance issues increase the risk of falls and injuries, especially in older persons. GLAV can also have an impact on social relationships and occupational performance, demanding a complete approach to ETD diagnosis and care to promote overall patient well-being.

4. Clinical presentation

4.1 Symptoms and signs

ETD typically presents a variety of symptoms, commonly acknowledged by otolaryngologists as muffled hearing, ear pain, tinnitus, decreased hearing, a sensation of fullness in the ears, and balance issues [14, 15]. However, GLAV, strongly associated with ETD, manifests a broader spectrum of symptoms that extend beyond the auditory system. These encompass gastrointestinal [11, 17, 20], autonomic [21, 22], and psychopathological aspects [19], including:

1. *Ear-related Symptoms:* Common symptoms include ear fullness or pressure, tinnitus, ear pain or headache, popping or clicking sensations, dizziness or balance problems, and ear itching.

2. *General Health and Well-Being:* Changes in sleep quality, appetite variations, fluctuations in energy levels, stress, and anxiety. Anxiety in GLAV patients specifically can stem from the fear of vertigo episodes, balance issues, and the unpredictability of symptoms.

3. *Gastrointestinal Disturbances and Laryngopharyngeal Reflux:* Nausea, vomiting, globus sensation (feeling of a lump in the throat), and hoarseness, which can be a symptom of laryngopharyngeal reflux, potentially secondary to ETD.

4. *Autonomic Responses:* Bradycardia (slow heart rate), respiratory difficulties, sweating episodes, and blood pressure changes.

5. *Psychopathological Aspects:* Heightened anxiety due to vestibular dysfunction, fear of falling or losing balance, avoidance behaviors, and the feedback loop between anxiety and vestibular symptoms.

6. *Cognitive and Behavioral Mechanisms:* Disorientation, postural instability, attentional and cognitive load issues influencing balance and orientation perception.

4.2 Diagnosis

Recognizing the extensive and varied symptoms associated with GLAV and ETD is essential for correct diagnosis and effective management, emphasizing the need for an integrated approach to patient care. The diagnostic process typically begins with otoscopy, tympanometry, and nasal endoscopy in a secondary care setting to evaluate the ear and nasopharyngeal areas [15].

5. Diagnostic criteria and methods for GLAV

Diagnosing GLAV needs a multidisciplinary approach, focusing on ETD and its impact on vestibular functions. The key goal in diagnostics is achieving balanced MEPs, ideally "0 daPa and 0 daPa," to accurately assess the vestibular symptoms specific to GLAV.

5.1 Clinical assessment

A comprehensive clinical assessment is required to diagnose and manage GLAV. This evaluation consists of the following components:

1. *Medical History review:* A comprehensive assessment of the patient's medical history is performed, with emphasis on the onset, duration, and particular characteristics of vertigo and any accompanying symptoms. This includes looking into any ear infections, surgeries, or Ear, Nose, and Throat (ENT) issues in the past. The assessment also considers the patient's exposure to environmental factors that may impact ear pressure.

2. *The physical examination*: Otoscopy is used to check for any abnormalities in the ear canal and tympanic membrane. Nasopharyngoscopy is used to evaluate the opening of the ET and look for evidence of NPR. Laryngoscopy is used to detect LPR. A neurological examination, with a special emphasis on the vestibulocochlear nerve, is required to determine whether the patient's symptoms are caused by a neurological condition.

5.2 Diagnostic testing

5.2.1 PTA

PTA is an essential diagnostic method for assessing hearing levels, especially in situations of GLAV. The study focuses on both low- and high-frequency hearing losses, with each providing distinct diagnostic insights:

1. *Low-Frequency Hearing Loss:* This is an indication of ETD, in which negative MEP leads to tympanic membrane retraction. Such retraction alters the ear's response to low-frequency sounds, indicating the presence of ETD.

2. *High-Frequency Hearing Loss:* Although rare, high-frequency hearing loss can indicate more chronic or severe ETD. This could be related to problems such as middle ear effusion, which hinders high-frequency sound transmission.

3. *Clinical Implications in GLAV:* It is crucial to identify these specific patterns of hearing loss when diagnosing ETD in the context of GLAV. Understanding the type and extent of hearing loss not only helps to confirm the ETD diagnosis, but it also helps to understand how ETD affects vestibular symptoms. This information is critical for building an effective treatment plan that is tailored to the needs of the person who is receiving treatment.

5.2.2 Tympanometry

Traditional tympanogram categories (A, Ad, As, B, and C) are insufficient for GLAV diagnosis. They need a more refined interpretation to detect minor ETD relevant to GLAV. Any variation from the "0 daPa and 0 daPa" norm suggests ETD, a significant part in GLAV, needing careful tympanometry investigation.

To summarize, tympanometry for GLAV necessitates a move from standard classifications and "within normal limits" to a focused examination on setting up balanced MEPs, ensuring exact diagnosis and effective GLAV care.

5.2.3 VFTs

Caloric Testing, Vestibular Evoked Myogenic Potentials (VEMP), Posturography, Videonystagmography (VNG), Rotational Chair Testing, Head Impulse Test (HIT), and Computerized Dynamic Posturography (CDP) are important VFTs for diagnosing GLAV and developing treatment options. Accurate test results require balanced MEPs.

1. *Caloric Testing:* Asymmetric MEPs can interfere with thermal stimuli conduction, potentially leading to false signs of unilateral vestibular weakness.

2. *VEMP:* Changes in MEP can affect sound transmission and thus test results.

3. *Rotary Chair Test:* While less directly influenced, considerable pressure changes can alter motion perception and results in the rotary chair test.

4. *Electronystagmography (ENG) /Videonystagmography (VNG):* Asymmetric MEPs can similarly affect the outcomes of these components.

5. *HIT and CDP:* Variations in MEP can have a direct impact on the results of the HIT and CDP, potentially changing balance and vestibular response evaluations due to MEP imbalances.

Given the dynamic nature of MEP, which is influenced by factors such as ET function and respiratory circumstances, getting a precise 0 daPa of MEP for VFTs can be difficult. In such cases, ETC is a useful technique. ETC provides a more direct method of managing and controlling MEP, potentially allowing for a closer approach to the ideal 0 daPa aim. This strategy is especially useful in situations when standard treatments fail, such as when there are considerable variations in MEP or ETD. ETC can thus improve VFT precision by ensuring that MEP is set as precisely as feasible to optimize test accuracy [14, 18].

5.3 Patient reported outcome measures (PROMs)

Utilizing PROMs that cover a wide array of symptoms, including those related to gastrointestinal [11, 17, 20], autonomic [21, 22], and psychopathological symptoms [19], can supply a deeper insight into the patient's condition.

5.4 ET function examination

Dr. Charles Bluestone's groundbreaking research emphasized the importance of ET function tests in diagnosing GLAV, particularly in patients with symptoms of ETD such as vertigo despite an intact tympanic membrane and no otitis media [12].

Based on personal insights, ET function testing with ETC and Toynbee diagnostic tube is advised even when PTA and impedance audiometry (IA) show normal results [14, 18]. Beyond the insights provided by Bluestone, this technique aids in thoroughly tackling the complexities of GLAV.

In GLAV instances, the incorporation of expanded testing ensures a thorough assessment for probable underlying ETD, leading to more correct diagnoses and effective treatment solutions.

The field of otolaryngology is evolving, with increased testing procedures reflecting a stronger understanding of GLAV and ETD. Bluestone's contributions continue to be a cornerstone of this continuing research, which is critical to improving patient care.

5.5 Imaging studies

Supportive tools like CT scans and MRIs are used to rule out other causes of vestibular symptoms that might mimic GLAV.

5.6 Reflux assessment

In the diagnostic process for GLAV, assessing reflux-related contributions to ETD is a crucial aspect. This involves two primary methods: pH monitoring and laryngoscopy. Both pH monitoring and laryngoscopy are vital for deciding whether reflux plays a role in a patient's ETD and consequent GLAV symptoms. Finding and treating underlying reflux conditions can be a key part in the effective management of GLAV, as controlling reflux may alleviate some of the ETD symptoms and improve overall ear and vestibular health [20].

5.7 Diagnostic criteria

The diagnosis of GLAV is based on criteria that link vestibular symptoms with ETD, with the primary goal of attaining a "0 daPa and 0 daPa" balanced MEP in both ears. This balance is critical for correctly diagnosing GLAV because it helps to rule out other potential causes of vestibular symptoms that are not related to ETD, assuring that the symptoms are caused by ETD-related difficulties.

1. *Vestibular Symptom Evaluation:* Initially, dizziness is assessed with a focus on diagnosing GLAV, with particular attention paid to symptoms at ground level and environmental pressure fluctuations.

2. *ETD Evaluation:* The presence of ETD, characterized by unequal MEP, is critical in the diagnosis of GLAV. To determine pressure balance, ETC is recommended.

3. *Equilibrium of MEP:* The achievement of "0 daPa and 0 daPa" in both ears is critical for GLAV diagnosis, distinguishing ETD-related symptoms from other VD. The importance of tympanometry in validating this balanced state cannot be overstated.

5.8 Differential diagnosis

The differential diagnosis of GLAV requires a multifaceted approach, incorporating assessments like alongside balanced MEP evaluation, laryngoscopy, nasopharyngoscopy, and the application of specialized PROMs. This comprehensive method is crucial for accurately distinguishing GLAV from other VD.

1. *Balanced MEP Evaluation:* Setting up equilibrium in MEP at "0 daPa and 0 daPa" is critical for differentiating GLAV from other vestibular conditions. This involves tympanometry and ET function tests to find the absence of ETD-related factors contributing to vestibular symptoms.

2. *Nasopharyngoscopy:* This diagnostic procedure examines the nasopharyngeal area and the ET opening. It is essential for finding structural or inflammatory issues that might mimic or contribute to vestibular symptoms, aiding in differentiating GLAV from other conditions.

3. *Laryngoscopy:* Given the reciprocal relationship between ETD and LPR, laryngoscopy is a vital part of the differential diagnosis. It helps in finding LPR, which can worsen or mimic symptoms of ETD and thus influence the presentation of GLAV [23].

4. *Application of New PROMs or ePROMs:* The use of newly developed PROMs, specifically designed for GLAV and ETD, is integral. These tools capture a broad spectrum of symptoms beyond the typical vestibular ones, for the exact diagnosis ETD. This wider symptom capture enables a more correct differentiation of GLAV from other vestibular disorders.

6. Management and treatment of GLAV

Understanding the reciprocal causal link between ETD and LPR is essential for effectively treating GLAV. GLAV, which causes vertigo owing to MEP imbalances, is frequently associated with these disorders. Normalization of MEP is critical in breaking the reciprocal cycle between ETD and LPR in GLAV management. In this scenario, ETC is important. ETC can help attenuate the influence of LPR on ET by directly intervening to rectify ETD, hence decreasing GLAV symptoms. In this therapy paradigm, effective LPR management through food, lifestyle changes, and medication is critical. Controlling LPR helps to lessen its aggravating effect on ETD, which aids in the management of GLAV symptoms [18, 20].

To reduce inflammation and improve ET function, pharmacological therapies such as decongestants, antihistamines, vasoconstrictors, mucolytics, antibiotics, and steroids are used. These medications address the ETD component of the cycle, hence influencing the effects of LPR indirectly [15].

Another method used in this comprehensive therapeutic strategy is balloon tuboplasty. It focuses on removing physical obstructions from the ET. The Valsalva technique, contrary to popular belief, is not indicated in postoperative care due to its potential dangers. Alternative procedures like ETC are recommended to ensure patient safety while retaining the procedure's efficacy [14].

If balance problems persist, vestibular rehabilitation is advised, pending normalization of middle ear pressures. This technique is designed to correct balance issues without exacerbating vertigo symptoms.

This therapeutic technique prioritizes patient education and support. Understanding GLAV, ETD, and LPR, as well as their interconnections, enables patients to engage in successful self-management strategies. In conclusion, GLAV management and treatment require a comprehensive approach that acknowledges and treats the reciprocal interaction between ETD and LPR. ETC, pharmaceutical therapies, balloon tuboplasty, and a comprehensive approach to LPR management all help to interrupt this complex loop and provide relief from GLAV symptoms [20].

7. Case studies and clinical evidence of GLAV

7.1 Illustrative case studies

7.1.1 Case study 1: chronic GLAV in a middle-aged adult: Meniere disease

Background: A 45-year-old female patient, a few years ago, experienced intermittent ear fullness and tinnitus, frequent coughing and chronic vertigo episodes. Initially misdiagnosed with Meniere's disease, surgery was suggested in a university hospital. She had nausea and prolonged tinnitus after intratympanic steroid injections. By the last year, the patient's gastrointestinal problems had worsened, and symptoms had spread to include stomach pain, flank pain, urine discomfort, and reflux esophagitis. The patient's habit of sniffing is indicative of chronic GLAV.

Clinical Assessment: During the initial clinic visit on December 2023, tympanometric measurements revealed severe negative pressures of −250 daPa in left ear and −7 aPa in the right, indicating ETD. This asymmetry in MEPs was suspected to be the source of the vestibular symptoms. Hearing difficulty and tinnitus were confirmed by audiometric tests, while gastroenterological investigations indicated gallstones and reflux esophagitis.

Intervention: ETC was used to manage the ETD due to the complex symptom profile and tympanometric results. Concurrently, the patient's gastrointestinal issues were treated.

Outcome: Post-catheterization, the patient reported significant alleviation of vertigo, confirmed by balanced middle ear pressures in follow-up tympanometry. Tinnitus was reduced, and episodes of ear fullness were eliminated. Additionally, the tailored therapy alleviated gastrointestinal problems. The patient currently reports no problems, indicating the ETC's efficacy in controlling the patient's illness.

This example demonstrates the efficacy of ETC in the treatment of GLAV, especially in complex patients with many symptoms and considerable asymmetric negative middle ear pressures. It emphasizes the significance of a thorough clinical evaluation and a multidisciplinary approach to treatment.

7.1.2 Case study 2: acute GLAV episode in a young adult: Otolithiasis

Background: A 30-year-old male, previously diagnosed with otolithiasis, experienced sudden dizziness and balance issues after a workout. Regularly drinking water before lying down, the patient was recommended to perform an Epley's maneuver technique by another otolaryngologist.

Clinical Assessment: Otoscopic examination was normal, but tympanometry revealed a notable MEP differential with negative pressures of −73 daPa in the left ear and −45 daPa in the right, indicating ETD.

Intervention: Following ineffective nasal decongestant use, ETC was successfully administered.

Outcome: Immediate symptom relief was noted post-procedure, with maintained ear pressure balance and no recurring vertigo in later follow-ups.

7.1.3 Case study 3: recurrent GLAV in an elderly person

Background: A 65-year-old male with a history of recurrent vertigo episodes that were initially misdiagnosed as age-related vestibular deterioration. The patient described episodes in response to weather changes and trouble adjusting to elevation variations when traveling.

Clinical Evaluation: Audiometric testing revealed a modest high-frequency hearing loss. Tympanometry revealed a negative −43 daPa MEP in the left ear and 0 daPa in the right eat, indicating ETD. Vestibular function tests found minor irregularities.

Intervention: A combination of ETC and vestibular rehabilitation activities, as well as dietary changes for mild LPR, were commenced.

Outcome: The patient reported a significant decrease in vertigo frequency and intensity, as well as improved tympanometry readings, indicating efficient ETD therapy.

7.1.4 Case study 4: GLAV in a teenager with allergic rhinitis

Background: A 17-year-old female with allergic rhinitis presented with episodes of dizziness and instability, particularly during allergy season. Initially unsuccessfully treated for benign paroxysmal positional vertigo (BPPV).

Clinical Assessment: Allergy testing revealed considerable nasal congestion. Tympanometry revealed a flat B type without middle ear effusion with unmeasurable MEP in the right ear and a positive 111 daPa MEP in the left ear, whereas VFTs were inconclusive due to changing results.

Intervention: Treatment included nasal steroids for allergic rhinitis and ETC sessions for ETD. Vestibular rehabilitation was postponed until MEP normalization.

Outcome: After several weeks, the patient reported a considerable decrease in vertigo occurrences, which correlated with improved tympanometric readings and reduced nasal symptoms.

7.2 Introduction of the article

> *A Case Report on Ground-Level Alternobaric Vertigo Due to Eustachian Tube Dysfunction with the Assistance of Conversational Generative Pre-Trained Transformer (ChatGPT) [24]*

Kim H (March 28, 2023) A Case Report on Ground-Level Alternobaric Vertigo Due to Eustachian Tube Dysfunction with the Assistance of Conversational Generative Pre-Trained Transformer (ChatGPT). Cureus 15(3): e36830. doi:10.7759/cureus.36830

This Dr. Hee-Young Kim's article supplies a comprehensive study on GLAV due to ETD, underscoring the necessity of correct diagnosis and effective interventions, such as ETC [24].

7.3 Additional reference

7.3.1 "Alternobaric vertigo: asymmetrical vestibular function due to asymmetrical middle ear pressures (Iron Man's Archenemy)"

Kim HY. Alternobaric vertigo: Asymmetrical vestibular function due to asymmetrical middle ear pressures (Iron Man's archenemy). [Internet]. ENT & Audiology News. Pinpoint Scotland Ltd; 2021 [cited 2023 Dec 13]. Available from: https://cloud.3dissue.net/30176/30070/30342/63730/index.html?page=42.

In this article, Dr. Hee-Young Kim discusses ABV, a result of asymmetrical vestibular function due to unequal middle ear pressures, emphasizing the importance of recognizing and managing ETD to effectively treat ABV. The article advocates for ETC as a crucial diagnostic and therapeutic tool in such cases [13].

7.3.2 "Eustachian tube catheterization: fundamental skill for competent otolaryngologists"

Kim HY. Eustachian tube catheterization: fundamental skill for competent otolaryngologists. *Journal of Otolaryngology ENT Research*. 2019;11(1):15–17. DOI: 10.15406/joentr.2019.11.00401

Dr. Hee-Young Kim's document highlights the critical role of ETC in diagnosing and treating ETD. The article delves into common symptoms, the technique of ETC, its diagnostic and therapeutic values, and the association between LPR/GERD and ETD, advocating ETC as an essential skill for otolaryngologists in managing ETD-related symptoms [18].

8. Modern perspectives and advances

This section examines recent advances in GLAV research and therapy, focusing on the integration of technology and patient-centered approaches.

8.1 The emerging role of biomarkers in GLAV diagnosis and management

In recent years, the possibility of identifying accurate biomarkers has opened up new paths in the diagnosis and treatment of GLAV. Biomarkers hold the promise of providing more objective, quantifiable measurements of disease prevalence and severity, potentially leading to earlier detection and more customized treatment regimens. While research on specific GLAV biomarkers is ongoing, the incorporation of such diagnostics offers significant promise for increasing our understanding of the condition and patient care. The identification and validation of these biomarkers such as middle ear pressure may alter the clinical approach to managing ETD and its related GLAV as the science progresses.

8.2 Mobile eye movement recording technology in vertigo diagnosis

Mobile eye movement recording technology, which enables real-time data capture during vertigo episodes, is a recent breakthrough. This approach is compatible with the recommendation for first ET function tests, resulting in more accurate diagnosis and aligning with modern diagnostic practices. Although the ET function test findings are unknown prior to the mobile eye movement recording test, data on eye movements during vertigo can be collected.

8.3 Development of new PROMs for ETD

A new PROMs instrument is being developed to evaluate the outcomes of ETC and other ETD therapies. The instrument intends to cover a wide variety of ETD symptoms, including gastrointestinal, autonomic, and psychopathological features, to improve the evaluation of treatment efficacy and patient quality of life [25]. The advancement entails: 1. Question formulation and refinement based on patient and expert feedback. 2. First clinical testing and evaluation of reliability and validity. Once completed, this PROM will be used in clinical practice for ETC patients and will be updated on a regular basis to reflect new findings and patient experiences. This technology will be crucial in improving ETD therapy and patient care.

8.4 electronic patient-reported outcome measures (ePROMs): a digital health initiative for ETD

The ePROMs program solves ETD's diagnostic shortcomings. It proposes a web-based tool for ETD management, with the goal of increasing patient interaction and standardizing outcome measurement. The effort forms smartphone apps and wearable devices for symptom monitoring, emphasizing the importance of digital health technology in ETD care.

These advances in GLAV diagnosis and treatment represent a move toward more precise, patient-centered approaches that incorporate technological improvements to improve care quality and patient outcomes [26].

9. Challenges and controversies

9.1 Current diagnosis and treatment obstacles

Diagnosis of GLAV poses special problems, particularly in emergency and outpatient settings. In emergency rooms, evaluating MEP is often disregarded, resulting in missed GLAV diagnoses. Delayed consultations following acute symptoms in outpatient clinics might make diagnosis GLAV challenging, as vestibular abnormalities may not be present during examination. An ideal diagnosis method would include testing as soon as symptoms appear.

9.2 Controversial issues and diverging points of view

Several disputed concerns continue in the study of GLAV. The pathogenesis remains unclear specifically how ETD causes GLAV and how it interacts with laryngopharyngeal reflux. Medical practitioners have yet to agree on MEP thresholds and the use of audiometry and tympanometry in diagnosing the condition. The methods of treatment are also contentious, with little agreement on the most effective interventions, including the importance of ETC. Managing patients presents its own set of issues, as doctors strive to combine acute symptom relief with long-term management goals, all within the context of personalized treatment. Focused research targeted at generating consistent recommendations is vital for advancing understanding and improving patient outcomes.

10. Identifying the key contributions of our GLAV

This chapter outlined the distinct features of GLAV in connection to ETD, emphasizing the importance of minor pressure variations at ground level. Accurate diagnosis is critical, requiring a systematic strategy to balancing MEP and applying a variety of treatments ranging from pharmaceuticals to vestibular rehabilitation to alleviate symptoms.

Advances in diagnostic procedures, personalized treatment plans, and the use of emerging technologies indicate substantial progress in the treatment of GLAV. A better understanding of its pathogenesis, as well as the development of prevention interventions, is required. Furthermore, comprehensive patient education initiatives and collaborative research activities are critical in moving this subject forward.

It is essential to reassess past and recent cases of vertigo for diagnostic accuracy. The use of tympanometry into diagnostic reports for vertigo patients is a crucial opportunity for improved GLAV identification, although its potential is underutilized. A determined attempt to systematically incorporate tympanometric evaluations—and to revisit earlier cases that may lack such data—can result in a reevaluation of diagnoses, encouraging a more detailed understanding of VD. This rigorous refinement of diagnostic methods is critical to the advancement of otolaryngology and the improvement of patient care.

The addition of rigorous diagnostic assessments, such as tympanometry, is critical in the progression of GLAV research. Updating diagnosis, both historical and current, will improve our understanding and the quality of care provided to patients suffering from vertigo-related conditions. Accepting these breakthroughs is critical to the ongoing improvement of otolaryngological treatments and patient health.

Conflict of interest

The author declares no conflict of interest.

Author details

Hee-Young Kim
Center for Executive and Continuing Professional Education at Harvard T.H. Chan School of Public Health, Boston, MA, USA

*Address all correspondence to: hee-young.kim-2022@ppcr.org

References

[1] Bluestone CD, Swarts JD, Furman JM, Yellon RF. Persistent alternobaric vertigo at ground level. The Laryngoscope. 2012;**122**:868-872. DOI: 10.1002/lary.22182

[2] Tjernström O. Alternobaric Vertigo. An Experimental Study in Man of Vertigo due to Atmospheric Pressure Changes [thesis]. Malmo, Sweden: Malmo General Hospital; 1974

[3] Lundgren CE. Alternobaric vertigo – A diving hazard. British Medical Journal. 1965;**2**:511-513. DOI: 10.1136/bmj.2.5460.511

[4] Deleau N. Des effets pathologiques de quelques lésions de l'oreille moyenne sur les muscles de l'expression faciale, sur l'organe de la vue et sur l'encephale. Paris: Delanchy; 1837. pp. 20-21

[5] Mudry A. History of Otology: A Tribute to Adam Politzer. Piribebuy, Paraguay: Wayenborgh; 2015

[6] Politzer A. Beiträge zur Physiologie des Gehörorgans. Sitzungsberichte der Kaiserlichen Akademie der Wissenschaften. 1861;**43**:427-438

[7] Mudry A. Adam Politzer (1835-1920) et la trompe d'Eustache [Adam Politzer (1835-1920) and the Eustachian tube]. Ann Otolaryngol Chir Cervicofac. 2004;**121**(2):75-82. DOI: 10.1016/s0003-438x (04)95493-x

[8] Mudry A. Josef Gruber (1827-1900) an underestimated Viennese Otologist in the shadow of Adam Politzer. Historical Otorhinolaryngology. 2015;**1**:21-29. Available from: https://www.historiaorl.com/wp-content/uploads/2015/04/Mudry-Weir-Gruber-and-Politzer.pdf

[9] Yearsley J. Deafness Practically Illustrated: Being an Exposition of the Nature, Causes and Treatment of Diseases of the Ear. London: John Churchill; 1863

[10] Allen P. Lectures on Aural Catarrh: Or, The Commonest Forms of Deafness and Their Cure. London: Churchill; 1871

[11] Merica FW. Vertigo due to obstruction of the Eustachian tubes. Journal of American Medical Association. 1942;**118**(15):1282-1284

[12] Bluestone CD. Eustachian Tube: Structure, Function, and Role in Middle-Ear Disease. 2e Kindle ed. Raleigh, North Carolina: People Medical Publishing House USA; 2018

[13] Teixeira MS. Understanding Eustachian tube function. Brazilian Journal of Otorhinolaryngology. 2020;**86**:523-524. DOI: 10.1016/j.bjorl.2020.02.001

[14] Kim HY. Alternobaric Vertigo: Asymmetrical Vestibular Function due to Asymmetrical Middle Ear Pressures (Iron Man's Archenemy). ENT & Audiology News. Pinpoint Scotland Ltd; 2021 [cited 2023 Dec 13]. Available from: https://cloud.3dissue.net/30176/30070/30342/63730/index.html?page=42

[15] Llewellyn A, Norman G, Harden M, Coatesworth A, Kimberling D, Schilder A, et al. Interventions for adult Eustachian tube dysfunction: A systematic review. Health Technology Assessment. 2014;**18**(46):1-180

[16] Schilder A, Bhutta M, Butler C, et al. Eustachian tube dysfunction: consensus statement on definition, types, clinical

presentation and diagnosis. Clinical Otolaryngology. 2015;**40**:407-411. DOI: 10.1111/coa.12475

[17] Kim H-Y. Vertigo due to Eustachian tube dysfunction. Archives of Otorhinolaryngology-Head & Neck Surgery. 2017;**1**(1):5. DOI: 10.24983/scitemed.aohns.2017.00017

[18] Kim H-Y. Eustachian tube catheterization: fundamental skill for competent otolaryngologists. Journal of Otolaryngology-ENT Research. 2019;**4**:11. DOI: 10.15406/joentr.2019.11.00401

[19] Yardley L. Overview of psychologic effects of chronic dizziness and balance disorders. Otolaryngologic Clinics of North America. 2000;**33**(3):603-616. DOI: 10.1016/s0030-6665(05)70229-2

[20] Kim H-Y. Reciprocal causal relationship between laryngopharyngeal reflux and Eustachian tube obstruction. Journal of Otolaryngology-ENT Research. 2015;**2**(6):195-198. DOI: 10.15406/joentr.2015.02.00046

[21] Thompson TL, Amedee R. Vertigo: A review of common peripheral and central vestibular disorders. The Ochsner Journal. 2009;**9**(1):20-26

[22] Sánchez-Manso JC, Varacallo M, Gujarathi R. Autonomic Dysfunction. StatPearls; 2022 Available from: https://www.ncbi.nlm.nih.gov/books/NBK430888/

[23] Park JJ, Luedeke I, Luecke K, Emmerling O, Westhofen M. Eustachian tube function in patients with inner ear disorders. European Archives of Oto-Rhino-Laryngology. 2013;**270**:1615-1621. DOI: 10.1007/s00405-012-2143-z

[24] Kim H-Y. A case report on ground-level alternobaric vertigo due to eustachian tube dysfunction with the assistance of conversational generative pre-trained Transformer (ChatGPT). Cureus. 2023;**15**(3):e36830. DOI: 10.7759/cureus.36830

[25] Group FNBW. Validation [Internet]. Food and Drug Administration (US); 2020 [cited 2023 Mar 1]. Available from: https://www.ncbi.nlm.nih.gov/books/NBK464453/

[26] Rosenberg SS, Carson BB, Kang A, Lee TH, Pandey R, Rizzo EJ. The Impact of Digital Health Technologies on Health Equity: Designing Research to Capture Patient-Reported Outcomes. Value and Outcomes Spotlight. ISPOR—The Professional Society for Health Economics and Outcomes Research. 2023 [cited 2023 Dec 18]. Available from: https://www.ispor.org/publications/journals/value-outcomes-spotlight/vos-archives/issue/view/addressing-assessment-and-access-issues-for-rare-diseases/the-impact-of-digital-health-technologies-on-health-equity-designing-research-to-capture-patient-reported-outcomes

Chapter 3

Impairment of Quality of Life after Temporal Bone Fractures

Elias Antoniades

Abstract

Temporal bone fractures (TBF) represent 14–22% of cranial fractures. The temporal bone is the thickest bone in the body, requiring excessive force to fracture; a TBF may occur in fresh human cadavers, when the applied force to the lateral skull is about 6000–8000 Newtons (equivalent to 600–800 Kilograms-force), increasing the risk of neurovascular injury. Conventionally, TBFs are categorized into longitudinal, transverse, and mixed types, depending on the direction of the fracture line. The complications of TBF include facial nerve palsy (FP), audiovestibular dyfunction, and cerebrospinal fluid (CSF) leak. All these sequels of TBFs may adversely affect the quality of life (QOL) with a psychological, emotional, and social impact. To our knowledge, the number of studies referring to QOL in patients suffering from TBF are very restricted. In this chapter, we elaborate on patient-assessed outcomes following TBF in relation to audiovestibular symptoms, apart from FP in adjunct with neurophysiological tests. Our aim to describe their impact on patients' QoL.

Keywords: temporal bone fracture, quality of life, facial palsy, hearing loss, dizziness

1. Introduction

Traumatic brain injuries (TBI) are caused by either a mild or severe hit of the cranium or in the context of penetrating injuries, as well [1]. TBIs are the etiology of long-term handicap for both children and adolescents. Approximately 40% of these groups warrants state financial aid [2]. Skull base fractures include the injury of significant neurovascular structures. These can occur either after a direct or indirect head blast [3]. They appear in the setting of motor vehicle accidents and falls [4]. The incidence of temporal bone fractures (TBF) rates 3% among all close TBIs, and many of them evade the diagnosis [5].

They concern mostly male patients (88.5%), and their epicenter is the temporomastoid suture. Approximately 60% are longitudinal fractures. Their signs are bleeding from nose and ear, which rate 36 and 32.7%, respectively. Hearing loss occurs in 10% of the patients, and 8% of them suffer facial palsy (FP). Finally, in 8.2% of the cases, cerebrospinal fluid (CSF) leakage is noticed [6].

These fractures are thus associated with both short-term and long-term complications, which are not properly evaluated, even when the patients are discharged from hospital.

2. Brief anatomic data of temporal bone

Temporal bone comprises five segments. These are the squamosal, the petrosal, the tympanic, and mastoid bones along with the styloid process, as well.

Petrosal bone is similar to a triangular pyramid (**Figure 1**). Its apex lies medially and its basis laterally. Its superior surface constitutes the abutment of middle cranial fossa [7]. The posterior surface is actually a part of the posterior cranial fossa [7].

Squamosal bone is the largest segment. Petrosquamosal suture separates it from petrosal bone. Temporalis muscle and superior temporal artery lie on the lateral surface of squamosal bone [7, 8].

Mastoid segment with the prominent mastoid process constitutes the attachment point of sternocleidomastoid and longus capitis muscles. In its medial surface lies a deep sulcus, which harbors sigmoid sinus [8]. In the front of the sigmoid sinus osseous case lies stylomastoid foramen, through which the facial nerve (FN) exits the cranium [7].

Tympanic bone has three surfaces: the anterior, the posterior, and the inferior. All three of them are the margins of external acoustic meatus. Tympanosquamous and tympanomastoid suture separates tympanic bones from the former divisions [7]. Finally, it becomes distinct from petrosal bone by petrotympanical fissure.

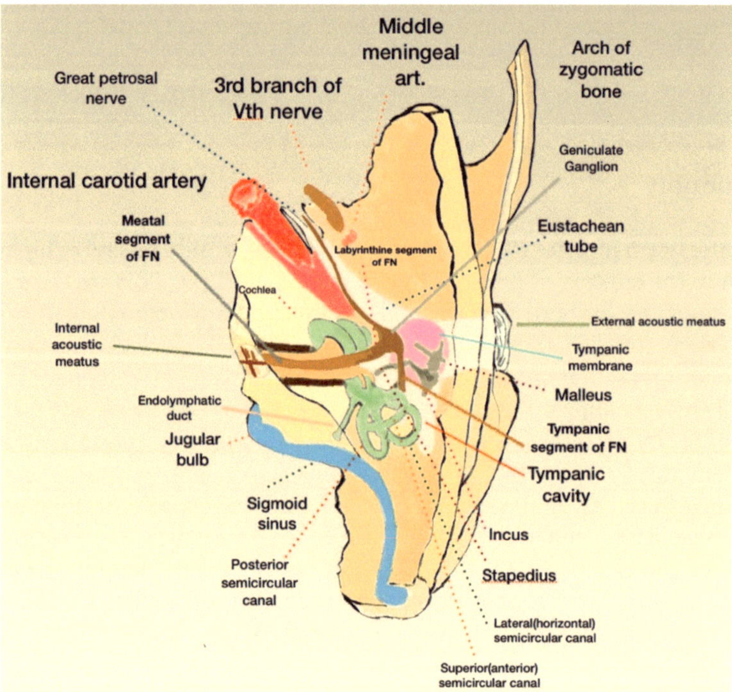

Figure 1.
Schematic representation of the most significant anatomical structures of a dissected right petrosal bone.

Styloid process is a marked spike projecting anteriorly and inferiorly. Its length is 3–4 cm. At its abutment, the stylomastoid foramen is localized [8].

3. Radiological classification of temporal bone fractures

Computer Tomography (CT) with thin slices was proven a sensitive method for the detection of TBFs [9]. CT-Angiography may be employed when the fracture line extends to the internal carotid foramen or toward the jugular foramen [10]. Based on the wide utilization of CT in TBIs, the first classifications of temporal bone fractures took place.

When the fracture's trajectory was parallel to the petrous bone axis, then the fractures were acknowledged as longitudinal ones [11]. Accordingly, when the trajectory was crossing this axis, we had the transverse fractures. There was also a third category, which was actually a combination of the aforementioned ones and were known as mixed fractures [11]. Longitudinal fractures constitute the majority (70–90%) of TBFs. They appear after a lateral blast at the parietotemporal area and are relevant with squamosal bone fractures [12]. When they originate from the mastoid tip or the posterior part of squama, they may reach foramen lacerum, invade tympanic cavity, break the osseous chain, and eventually transect the genu of the FN [11]. One fifth of the patients with longitudinal TBF manifest FP, which is mostly incomplete. In these cases, avulsion of great superficial petrosal nerve coexists (**Figure 2A**) [11].

Transverse fractures are less frequent and constitute one-third of TBFs. They occur after blast on the frontal or occipital areas. They are delineated between either jugularis foramen or foramen magnum and middle cranial fossa (**Figure 2B**) [12].

Recent classifications have focused on the violation of the otic capsule [13]. The non-violating fractures emerge from mastoid cells and cross the roof of tympanic cavity. They are linked with low rates of FP. They are responsible for hemotympanum and either conductive hearing loss (HL) or mixed one. The last one is caused by osseous chain breakage [14]. The violating fractures relate to CSF effusion and sensory HL. They may occasionally extend from petrosal pyramid to foramen magnum [14].

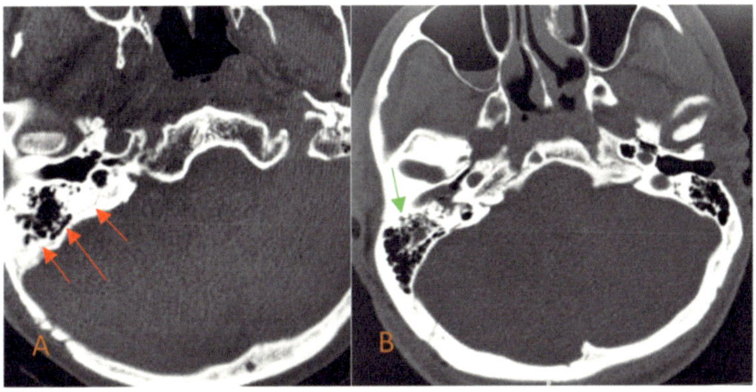

Figure 2.
A. Longitudinal TBF B. Transverse TBF. Both types may not exhibit significant distension and may easily misdiagnosed. Therefore, CT with very thin slices is necessary for TBF detection.

4. TBF sequels and their evaluation

4.1 Posttraumatic facial palsy (FP) and its evaluation

Due to the solid consistency of temporal bone, the severity of TBI is proportional to the fracturing force [15]. The initial assessment of FN function commences after patient's stabilization. Clinical signs, such as ear bleeding, mastoid process hematoma, tympanic membrane rupture, and disequilibrium or FP are strong indications for the employment of high-resolution CT [15].

Three clinical scenarios exist concerning FN injury. In the first case, the injury is the result of axonal swelling or localized hematoma. FP occurs late and may progress to paralysis. Outcome is overall favorable, and FP recurs completely in the majority of the patients [16]. In the second case, bone spicules compress the facial nerve. Therefore, FP has immediate onset and may be either complete or incomplete. Finally, the FN can be transected and surgical restoration is warranted. FP's outcome in this scenario is dismal [17].

Compared to the lower incidence of FP in longitudinal fractures, it is observed in almost half of the transverse fractures [18].

In longitudinal fractures, the labyrinthine segment of FN is injured in 60% of the cases [11]. In transverse fractures, this ratio is even greater counting 67% [19]. Labyrinthine segment of FN courses within the thinnest part of fallopian canal [19].

Categorization of the severity of peripheral FP is performed using the six-grade House–Brackmann scale [20]. Neurophysiological evaluation is an objective method of facial nerve functionality. This has to be performed at House-Brackmann [HB] grade III or more. HB I is considered as normal function, HB II as mild palsy, HB III-IV as moderate palsy, and HB V-VI as severe palsy, **Table 1** [20].

Electroneurography (ENoG) is performed between the 4th and 14th day and estimates the Wallerian degeneration [21]. It utilizes the maximal electrical stimulation to excite the extracranial FN. Superficial electrodes record the biphasic compound action potential of muscles, which depends on the simultaneous depolarization of active nerve axons [21]. Afterwards, a comparison with the healthy side is drawn.

House-Brackmann Scale			
Grade I-Normal	**Normal facial function**		
Grade II-Slight dysfunction	Forehead Moderate to good function	Eye Complete closure with minimum effort	Mouth Slight asymmetry
Grade III-Moderate dysfunction	Forehead Slight to moderate movement	Eye Complete closure with effort	Mouth Slightly weak with maximum effort
Grade IV-Moderate severe dysfunction	Forehead No movement	Eye Incomplete closure	Mouth Asymmetric with maximum effort
Grade V-Severe dysfunction	Forehead No movement	Eye Incomplete closure	Mouth Slight movement
Grade VI-Total paralysis	No movement		

Table 1.
House Brackmann Facial Nerve Function Grading [20].

Subsequently, the percentage of the degenerated axons is calculated [22]. Upon 14 days, degeneration reaches its zenith and patients who had not exhibited 90% degeneration or more do not warrant surgical procedure [23]. ENoG may be performed at regular follow-up periods [24].

Nerve excitability test is based on the principle that the prolonged depolarization of neurons increases their excitation. The examiner utilizes a probe that administrates electric current whose maximal intensity is 20 mA. In this test, a comparison between the two hemispheres of face is drawn, as well. Difference greater than 3,5 mA at excitation documentation signifies abnormal response [25].

4.2 Indications and types of surgical treatment

Labyrinthine segment and Geniculate Ganglion (GG) are the most frequently injured divisions of FN [26]. Neurapraxia recedes usually within one and a half month [12]. Both delayed and immediate paralysis should be initially observed. Complete or almost complete convalescence is noticed in the vast majority of both categories [4].

Surgical intervention is indicated in cases of immediate and highly severe palsy (House Brackman scale V or VI), which reveals either no responses in nerve excitability test or more than 95% degeneration in ENoG [18].

Decompression is usually performed within the first 14 days [27] and seldom upon the third month after the injury [28]. Apart from the severity of palsy, hearing function has to be co-evaluated. Finally, TBF trajectory and pertinent anatomy should be elaborated [27].

Transmastoid approach was at first performed in cases of longitudinal fractures, whose trajectory was along with the tympanic or mastoid division of FN and lateral to GG. It is a low-risk and efficacious surgery, which does not need craniotomy [29]. Tympanic division of FN and GG can be explored *via* the transmastoid approach. Its disadvantage is that the anterior semicircular canal with its ampulla restricts the preparation of the labyrinthine division of FN [30].

Middle fossa or translabyrinthine procedures are optimal for entire FN preparation co-estimating the auditory function. The middle fossa corridor confers exposure of the labyrinthine division and GG maintaining the current auditory function [23]. Hearing deficits, bleeding, ischemia, and leakage are rare but potential complications [31]. Translabyrinthine decompression yields further decompression to GG, as well. It can be applied in cases of severe hearing impairment. It encompasses drilling *via* the mastoid process and semicircular canals, providing access even to the internal acoustic meatus [30].

4.2.1 Hearing loss (HL) and its evaluation

HL can be conductive, sensorineural, or of mixed type. Conductive HL belongs to the short-term complications of TBF. Its incidence rates 58 and 27% in adult and pediatric population, respectively [32]. Hemotympanum is the commonest etiology and recurs almost always completely [32]. Other causes include the rupture of tympanic membrane, which is observed in longitudinal fractures [33] and has immediate onset [34]. Only one-fourth of the patients have symptoms after 6 weeks [35]. It is considered refractory when it persists more than 4 months. Luxation of osseous chain should be suspected, when hearing loss is greater than 30 dB. Incus is the most affected ossicle, and incostapedial luxation is the most frequent injury of ossicular chain [36].

Sensorineural HL after TBF is associated with cochlear hemorrhages, injury of Corti apparatus, or perilymphatic fistula, and its incidence is 14–23% [37].

Transverse fractures violate otic capsule and result in sensorineural HL. Stapedius base is afflicted, and later, perilymphatic fistula appears [38]. Acoustic nerve itself can also be directly injured [39]. Sensory HL appears in longitudinal fractures, as well. It is imputed to labyrinth concussion [39]. The severity of HL stabilizes within 12 months [40].

Tonic audiogram evaluates hearing function by using the responses of the examinee depending on the perception of specific sound tones. It also estimates air and bone conduction [41]. Air conduction assessment takes place between 125 Hz and 8 kHz, whereas bone conduction takes place between 250 Hz and 4 kHz. Speech discrimination test should always be included [41].

High frequency auditory dysfunction (3–6 kHz) corresponds to acoustic nerve avulsion and, subsequently, to sensorineural hearing loss [42].

Conversely, great discrepancy between air and bone conductivity-with maximal difference 65 dB- denotes conductivity HL [43].

4.2.2 Posttraumatic tinnitus

Tinnitus appears as a consequence of hearing ascending pathways dysfunction [44] and can be permanent when otic capsule is violated [44]. Its incidence varies from 4.9–53% in TBIs [45]. It is classified in pulsive and non-pulsive one. Non-pulsive is the most frequent type [46]. Tinnitus etiology involves not only cochlear impairment [47] but also ascending pathways excess activation, as it was mentioned above [48].

The great discrepancy in its incidence can be attributed to the deficient report from patients' side and to its underestimation by treating physicians. Hyperacousis usually coexists. The majority of the sufferers are young males [45]. Its intensity exacerbates with oculomotion, light touch, and involuntary muscular contractions [49]. Tonic audiogram has a diagnostic role, inasmuch as tinnitus is detected among the high frequencies [45].

4.2.3 Posttraumatic vertigo

Vertigo occurs after either immediate injury of membranous labyrinth and vestibule or after the formation of perilymphatic fistula. Finally, it may coexist with injury of the superior semicircular canal [50]. It is predominantly of peripheral type and is present in half of the patients who are not hospitalized [51]. One-fifth of the patients with TBI suffer their symptoms for at least 2 years [52].

Benign positional paroxysmal vertigo (BPPV) is the most frequent form of vestibular dysfunction, and one-third of patients suffer a refractory form [53, 54]. Its onset is late and usually appears unilaterally [55, 56].

4.2.4 Posttraumatic cerebrospinal fluid (CSF) leakage

Leptomeningeal rupture in the setting of TBF has as result the violation of. subarachnoid space and the outflow of CSF either through the ear or through the nose.

Otorrhoea is observed mostly in longitudinal fractures, when tegmentum ruptures. The onset can be either immediate or late [55]. TBFs with violated otic capsule also exhibit CSF leakage. Rhinorrhoea occurs, *via* the Eustachian tube. It may lead to bacterial meningitis. *Streptococcus pneumoniae*, Neisseria meningitides, and *Haemophilus influenzae* are the most common pathogens. The relative risk varies from 4 to 50% [56]. Meningitis may ensue even after years [57].

Half of the cases with CSF leakage recur by keeping the patients bedridden solely or by the placement a lumbar drainage [58]. Precautionary administration of antibiotics is not recommended [59]. When leakage persists more than 5 days, then surgical repair is warranted [60, 61]. The latter should be performed within 7 to 9 days [4].

5. Quality of life and its impairment in patients with TBF

5.1 Attempts of defining and estimating quality of life

Quality of life (QoL) is not a strict definition. In clinical praxis, the term health related quality of life is more usually encountered. The parameters that are encompassed in these definitions are the overall health status, physical and emotional function of the examinees, the deterioration of cognitive and sexual performance, and social extroversion. Therefore, there exist inventories that either evaluate the overall QoL or focus on some of these fields [62].

Patients tend to underestimate their handicaps, due to the variability of their severity during the time period of their disease or due to their adaptation to the new conditions. For this reason, these questionnaires have to be appraised together with objective clinical tools [63].

5.2 Impairment of quality of life

5.2.1 FP and patients' handicap

FP affects the daily function and the social interaction of individuals [64]. In studies, which assess the QoL, almost 75% of the patients with FP exhibit deterioration of their QoL. This is correlated with the severity of the FP either initially or at the end of the study period [65]. FP may, indeed, have impact on the results of social or emotional component of the inventories [66].

In fact, these patients tend to isolate, and they present an inhibition of their social behavior [67]. Volk et al. [68] evaluated the QoL in patient with both idiopathic and posttraumatic FP. Their study revealed that elder and female patients gave worse responses in the social/emotional parts of the inventories. They also found that the more severe the initial FP was the worst outcome of the physical scale was. Interestingly, as far as the physical components are concerned, only one-third of the patients with posttraumatic FP exhibited severe impairment [68].

In studies that evaluated the QoL after idiopathic FP, it was shown that majorly female patients tend to have worse outcome in the social/emotional parts [69]. Furthermore, it was documented that mixed fractures, as a combined pattern of forces, lead frequently to breakage [70] and consequently in FP [70]. One-fourth of these patients demonstrate worse outcome in social/emotional subscales [71, 72].

The immediate onset of the FP is not an indication of prompt surgical procedure, as long as decompression does not alter the course of the FP [16]. On the other hand, the late onset of FP is treated well with conservative methods [73].

ENoG and nerve excitability test are widely used for the prognosis of nerve restoration [74]. In ENoG, degeneration greater than 95% is considered ominous, especially within the first 14 days after the trauma [75]. Deterioration of physical aspects of QoL has been shown to be linked with marked degeneration [72]. Likewise, nerve excitability test results are a predictor of FP recovery [27]. Abnormal responses from both of these tests portend poor outcome in QoL [72].

5.2.2 HL, audiovestibular impairment, and patients' handicaps

5.2.2.1 HL and its impact on QoL

HL and tinnitus lead to poor communication, depression, and social isolation by deteriorating the QoL significantly, especially in the elderly [76]. Even in the unilateral profound HL with loss of speech discrimination, social activities are markedly hindered [77].

Mixed pattern of HL relates to worse outcome in audiogram examination [78]. This type of HL is implicated in the destruction of outer hair cell layer. This layer is responsible for the speech discrimination in noisy background [79].

Cochlear structural lesions induce the neuroplasticity process of central auditory pathways [80]. These alterations ignite a series of neuronal discharges and the occurrence of tinnitus [81]. This misperception is further amplified by posttraumatic stress [82]. Stressful impairment appears late, when the rest and more serious trauma sequels recede [45].

Disequilibrium and vertigo appear in almost 60% of patients who suffered TBI [83]. In cases of TBFs, this percentage reaches 67%. The characteristics of dizziness are these of BPPV [62]. The symptoms are self-recessing, and they dampen within 3 to 12 months [43].

5.2.2.2 Long term sequels of HL

HL is a contributor of cognitive decline and dementia. Approximately 35% of dementia cases can be prevented and avoided. HL constitutes one of the nine aggravating factors for dementia and is considered a reversible one [84]. Hearing impairment itself relates to cerebral atrophy and especially of the right temporal lobe [85]. Parallel studies have revealed that auditory dysfunction is associated with decreased cerebral volume [86]. Alternative hypotheses support that cognitive decline is not attributed directly to deficient hearing, but to the limited physical activity and social isolation [87].

Sometimes, patients report subjective symptoms of hearing after TBF [88, 89]. Kisilevski et al. [90] appraised the subjective hearing dysfunction and behavior. About 40% of their participants reported hearing difficulties, despite the normal results in their audiogram. Attias et al. [91] examined patients with mild and moderate TBIs and whose audiograms were normal. Interestingly, seven out of ten of them reported tinnitus, hindered speech discernment, and hyperacusis in slightly noisy ambience. Assumingly, the central processing of auditory cortex and the central compensation participate in the pathophysiology of this phenomenon [92]. The central compensation after cochlear injury may vary in its severity [93].

Another term that has to be discussed is the labyrinthine concussion. This term was initially used to describe labyrinthine lesions without TBF [94, 95]. In histopathologic studies, it is documented that the loss of hair cells and Scarpa's ganglion cells occur in the context of TBIs [96]. Inner ear bleeding, cochlear nerve avulsion, and blockage of endolymphatic duct were considered as potential causes [97]. This mechanism of local cochlear synaptopathy may corroborate the coexistence of tinnitus in case of hearing impairment [97].

5.2.2.3 Long-term sequels of audiovestibular dysfunction

Mild TBIs are associated with dizziness. Studies relevant with TBIs in sports reported that 55% of the patients claim dizziness [97]. The latter is actually the most common complaint in TBIs [98]. One-third of sufferers reported no improvement even after 2 weeks [99]. Paradoxically, no association was observed between the loss of consciousness after the trauma and the persistence of dizziness [100].

Apart from the medium-term sequels long-term signs, such as anxiety, depression and post-concussive syndrome exist. Their etiology is imputed to the interconnection of vestibulo-occular reflex pathway and vestibulospinal fascicle *via* brainstem, cerebellum, and frontal lobe [99].

Tinnitus perception is aggravated by the presence of dizziness. The inverse relationship was not proven, though [101]. Vestibular cues are significant for the storage of spatial information to hippocampus [101, 102]. According to studies with functional magnetic resonance imaging (fMRI), posterior insula, superior temporal gyrus, inferior parietal lobule, cingular gyrus, and precuneus contribute in this storage process, as well [103]. Therefore, vestibular dysfunction is relevant with impaired self-awareness and member misperception [104].

6. Conclusions

TBFs may occur in all forms of TBIs, namely, from mild to severe ones. Their consequences on QoL may emerge and endure in the long term and are frequently underestimated.

Post-traumatic FP has a significant impact on patients' physical function and social interaction. Despite the fact that the physical handicaps may recede, the psychosocial factors have to be addressed to optimize patients' satisfaction and QoL. Both the pattern of TBF, especially the mixed ones and the results of neurophysiological examinations, constitute prognostic factors. Thereby, cases with immediate onset and severely abnormal responses in either ENoG or excitability test can establish the prognosis.

Results of tonic audiogram and TBF type are prognosticators for the long-term audiovestibular outcome. Post-traumatic HL, tinnitus, and vestibular dysfunction in one or both ears may also lead to deficient communication, anxiety, and social withdrawal.

Not so seldom, the audiovestibular sequels of TBFs manifest common symptoms with post-concussive syndrome. Therefore, they may be considered a transient phenomenon, which is not the case.

Multimodal approach and regular follow-up controls by otolaryngologists, neurosurgeons, and psychologists are necessary for these patients.

Notes/thanks/other declarations

I would like to thanks Prof. Psillas G.of. 1st.Neurosurggical University ENT Clinic for his assistance and elaborate explanation of ENT diagnostic methods.

Author details

Elias Antoniades
Second Neurosurgical Clinic, Ippokrateion General Hospital, Thessaloniki, Greece

*Address all correspondence to: eliasantoniad@yahoo.gr

References

[1] Centers for Disease Control and Prevention. Surveillance Report of Traumatic Brain Injury-Related Emergency Department Visits, Hospitalizations, and Deaths. Atlanta, Georgia: Centers for Disease Control and Prevention, U.S. Department of Health and Human Services; 2014. Available from: https://www.cdc.gov/traumaticbraininjury/get_the_facts.html [Accessed: July 8, 2019]

[2] Eapen B, Cifu D. Rehabilitation after Traumatic Brain Injury. St. Louis (MO): Elsevier Inc.; 2018

[3] Brawley BW, Kelly WA. Treatment of basal skull fractures with and without cerebrospinal fluid fistulae. Journal of Neurosurgery. 1967;**26**:57-61

[4] Brodie HA, Thompson TC. Management of complications from 820 temporal bone fractures. The American Journal of Otology. 1997;**18**:188-197

[5] Patel A, Lofgren DH, Varacallo M. Temporal Fracture. Treasure Island, (FL): StatPearls Publishing; 2022

[6] Amin Z, Sayuti R, Kahairi A, Islah W, Ahmad R. Head injury with temporal bone fracture: One year review of case incidence, causes, clinical features and outcome. The Medical Journal of Malaysia. 2008;**63**(5):373-376

[7] Sanna M, Russo A, Taibah A. The Temporal Bone: Anatomical Dissection and Surgical Approaches. 1st ed. New York-Stutgart: Thieme; 2018

[8] Standring S. Gray's Anatomy E-book. 42nd ed. China: Elsevier; 2021

[9] Jackson G, Hamilton N, Tupler L. Detecting traumatic brain injury among veterans of operations enduring and Iraqi freedom. North Carolina Medical Journal. 2008;**69**:43-47

[10] Jones RM, Rothman MI, Gray WC, Zoarski GH, Mattox DE. Temporal lobe injury in temporal bone fractures. Archives of Otolaryngology – Head & Neck Surgery. 2000;**126**(2):131-135

[11] Cannon CR, Jahrsdoerfer RA. Temporal bone fractures. Review of 90 cases. Archives of Otolaryngology. 1983;**109**(5):285-288

[12] Darrouzet V, Duclos JY, Liguoro D, et al. Management of facial paralysis resulting from temporal bone fractures: Our experience in 115 cases. Otolaryngology and Head and Neck Surgery. 2001;**125**(1):77-84

[13] Schuknecht HF. Pathology of the Ear. Philadelphia, PA: Lea and Febiger; 1993

[14] Mantokoudis G, Schläpfer N, Kellinghaus M, et al. Traumatic dislocation of middle ear ossicles: A new computed tomography classification predicting hearing outcome. PLoS One. 2021;**16**(2):e0245796

[15] Gantz BJ. Traumatic Facial Paralysis, in Current Therapy in Otolaryngology Head and Neck Surgery. Hamilton, (ON): C Decker; 1987. pp. 112-115

[16] Nash JJ, Friedland DR, Boorsma KJ, et al. Management and outcomes of facial paralysis from intratemporal blunt trauma: A systematic review. Laryngoscope. 2010;**120**(7):1397-1404

[17] Ardhaoui H, Halily S, Abada R, Rouadi S, Roubal M, Mahtar M. Simultaneous bilateral traumatic facial palsy with different treatment protocols.

International Journal of Surgery Case Reports. 2020;**74**:66-68

[18] Aguilar EA, Yeakley JW, Ghorayeb BY, Hauser M, Cabrera J, Jahrsdoerfer RA. High-resolution CT-scan of temporal bone fractures- association of facial nerve paralysis with temporal bone fractures. Head & Neck Surgery. 1987;**9**:162-166

[19] Fisch U. Facial paralysis in fractures of petrous bone. Laryngoscope. 1974;**84**:2141-2154

[20] House JE, Brackmann DE. Facial nerve grading system. Otolaryngology and Head and Neck Surgery. 1985;**93**:146-147

[21] Fish U. Facial nerve grafting. Otolaryngologic Clinics of North America. 1974;**7**(2):517-529

[22] Krarup C. Compound sensory action potential in normal and pathological human nerves. Muscle & Nerve. 2004;**29**(4):465-483

[23] Fisch U. Surgery for Bell's palsy. Archives of Otolaryngology. 1981;**107**(1):1-11

[24] Liu Y, Han J, Zhou X, Gao K, Luan D, Xie F, et al. Surgical management of facial paralysis resulting from temporal bone fractures. Acta Oto-Laryngologica. 2014;**134**(6):656-660. DOI: 10.3109/00016489.2014.892214

[25] Nodera H, Kaji R. Nerve excitability testing and its clinical application to neuromuscular diseases. Clinical Neurophysiology. 2006;**117**(9):1902-1916

[26] Aslan H, Songu M, Eren E, Basoglu MS, Özkul Y, Ates D, et al. Results of decompression with middle cranial fossa approach or traumatic intratemporal fascial nerve injury. Journal of Craniofacial Surgery. 2014;**25**(4):1305-1308

[27] Chang CY, Cass SP. Management of facial nerve injury due to temporal bone trauma. The American Journal of Otology. 1999;**20**(1):96-114

[28] Quaranta A, Campobasso G, Piazza F, et al. Facial nerve paralysis in temporal bone fractures: Outcomes after late decompression surgery. Acta Oto-Laryngologica. 2001;**121**(5):652-655

[29] Gür H, Görür K, Ismi O, et al. Surgical outcomes of transmastoid facial nerve decompression for patients with traumatic facial nerve paralysis. The Journal of International Advanced Otology. 2021;**17**(4):294-300

[30] Yetiser S, Satar B, Kazkayasi M. Immunologic abnormalities and surgical experiences in recurrent facial nerve paralysis. Otology and Neurotology. 2002;**23**(5):772-778

[31] Weber PC, Gantz BJ. Results and complications from acoustic neuroma excision via middle cranial fossa approach. Otology & Neurotology. 1996;**17**(4):669-675

[32] Waissbbluth S, Ywakim R, Al Qassabbi B, et al. Pediatric temporal bone fractures: A case series. International Journal of Pediatric Otorhinolaryngology. 2016;**84**:106-109

[33] Grant JR, Arganbright J, Friedland DR. Outcomes for conservative management of traumatic conductive hearing loss. Otology & Neurotology. 2008;**29**(3):344-349

[34] Griffin JE, Altenau MM, Schaefer SD. Bilateral longitudinal temporal bone fractures: A retrospective review of seventeen cases. Laryngoscope. 1979;**89**:1432-1435

[35] Dommerby H, Tos M. Sensorineural hearing-loss in posttraumatic incus dislocation. Archives of Otolaryngology. 1983;**109**:257-261

[36] Nosan DKK, Benecke JE Jr, Murr AH. Current perspective on temporal bone trauma. Otolaryngology and Head and Neck Surgery. 1997;**117**(1):67-71

[37] Hough JVD. Otologic trauma. In: Paparella MM, Shumrick DA, editors. Otolaryngology. Vol. 2. Philadelphia, PA: W.B. Saunders; 1980. pp. 1656-1679

[38] Fitzgerald DC. Head trauma: Hearing loss and dizziness. The Journal of Trauma. 1996;**40**:488-496

[39] Dahiya R, Keller JD, Litofsky NS, Bankey PE, Bonassar LJ, Megerian CA. Temporal bone fractures: Otic capsule violating clinical and radiographic considerations. The Journal of Trauma. 1999;**47**:1079-1083

[40] Gentry L. Temporal bone trauma: Current perspectives for diagnostic evaluation. Neuroimaging Clinics of North America. 1991;**1**:319-340

[41] Segal, Samuel; Eviatar, Ephraim; Berenholz, Leonard; Kessler, Alexander; Shlamkovitch, Nathan dynamics of sensorineural hearing loss after head trauma, Otology & Neurotology 2002;23 (3): 312-315

[42] Peters RW, Moor BC, Baer T. Speech reception threshold in noise with and without spectral and temporal dips for hearing impaired and normally hearing people. The Journal of the Acoustical Society of America. 1998;**103**:577-587

[43] Cvorovic L, Jovanovic MB, Markovic M, Milutinovic Z, Strbac M. Management of complication from temporal bone fractures. European Archives of Oto-Rhino-Laryngology. 2012;**269**(2):399-403

[44] Rosowski JJ, Relkin EM. Introduction to analysis of middle- ear function. In: Jahn AF, Santos-Sacchi J, editors. Physiology of the Ear. 2nd ed. San Diego, CA: Singular; 2001

[45] Kim BJ, Song I, Choi J, Rah YC. Contralateral hearing loss in temporal bone fractures: A potential association with combined intracranial injury. The Journal of International Advanced Otology. 2024;**20**(3):210-215

[46] Kreuzer PM, Landgrebe M, Schecklmann M, Staudinger S, Langguth B. Trauma-associated tinnitus: Audiological, demographic and clinical characteristics. PLoS One. 2012;**7**:e45599

[47] Nicolas-Puel C, Faulconbridge RL, Guitton M, Puel JL, Mondain M, Uziel A. Characteristic of tinnitus and etiology of associated hearing loss: A study of 123 patients. The International Tinnitus Journal. 2002;**8**:37-44

[48] Moller AR. Pathophysiology of tinnitus. The American Journal of Otology. 1997;**18**:577-585

[49] Jannetta PJ. Observations on the etiology of trigeminal neuralgia, hemifacial spasm, acoustic nerve dysfunction, and glossopharyngeal neuralgia: Definitive microsurgical treatment and results in 117 patients. Acta Neurochirurgica. 1997;**20**:145-154

[50] Levine RA, Abel M, Cheng H. CNS somatosensory-auditory interactions elicit or modulate tinnitus. Experimental Brain Research. 2003;**153**(4):643-648

[51] Shea JJ Jr, Ge X, Orchik DJ. Traumatic endolymphatic hydrops. American Journal of Otolaryngology. 1995;**16**(2):235-240

[52] Kushner D. Mid traumatic brain injury: Toward understanding manifestations and treatment. Archives of Internal Medicine. 1998;**158**:1617-1624

[53] Vertigo BT. Its Multisensory Syndromes. London: Springer; 1999

[54] Friedman JM. Post-traumatic vertigo. Medicine and Health, Rhode Island. 2004;**87**(10):296-300

[55] Shepard NT. Balance and dizziness. In: Zasler ND, Katz DI, Zafonte RD, editors. Brain Injury Medicine: Principles and Practice. New York: Demos Medical Publishing; 2013. pp. 779-793

[56] Schuknecht HF. Cupulolithiasis. Archives of Otolaryngology. 1969;**90**:765-778

[57] Narayan RK. Head injury. In: Grossman RG, Hamilton WJ, editors. Principles of Neurosurgery. New York: Raven; 1991. pp. 235-291

[58] Nageris B, Hansen MC, Lavelle WG, Van Pelt FA. Temporal bone fractures. The American Journal of Emergency Medicine. 1995;**13**:211-214

[59] Ratilal BO, Costa J, Sampaio C, Papamikail L. Antibiotic prophylaxis for preventing meningitis in patients with basilar skull fractures. Cochrane Database of Systematic Reviews. 2011;**8**:CD004884

[60] Gosal J, Gurmey T, Kursa G, et al. Is acetazolamide really useful in the management of traumatic cerebrospinal fluid rhinorrhea? Neurology India. 2015;**63**(2):197-201

[61] Lo YL, Yang TC, Liao CC, Yang ST. Diagnosis of traumatic internal carotid artery injury: The role of craniofacial fracture. The Journal of Craniofacial Surgery. 2007;**18**(2):361-368

[62] Karnath HO, Dieterich M. Spatial neglect--a vestibular disorder? Brain. 2006;**129**(Pt 2):293-305

[63] Fayers PM, Machin D. Quality of Life the Assessment, Analysis and Reporting of Patient- Reported Outcomes. 3rd ed. West Sussex, UK: Willey Blackwell; 2015

[64] Ricciardiello F, Mazzone S, Longo G, Russo G, Piccirillo E, Sequino G, et al. Our experience on temporal bone fractures: Retrospective analysis of 141 cases. Journal of Clinical Medicine. 2021;**10**:201

[65] Montava M, Mancini J, Masson C, Collin M, Chaumoitre K, Lavieille JP. Temporal bone fractures: Sequelae and their impact on quality of life. American Journal of Otolaryngology. 2015;**36**: 364-370

[66] Van Swearingen JM, Cohn JF, Turnbull J, Mrzai T, Johnson P. Psychological distress: Linking impairment with disability in facial neuromotor disorders. Otolaryngology and Head and Neck Surgery. 1998;**118**:790-796

[67] Van den Elzen ME, Versnel SL, Hovius SE, Passchier J, Duivenvoorden HJ, Mathijssen IM. Adults with congenital or acquired facial disfigurement: Impact of appearance on social functioning. Journal of Cranio-Maxillo-Facial Surgery. 2012;**40**:777-782

[68] Volk GF, Granitzka T, Kreysa H, Klingner CM, Guntinas-Lichius O. Initial severity of motor and non-motor disabilities in patients with facial palsy: An assessment using patient-reported outcome measures. European Archives of Oto-Rhino-Laryngology. 2017;**274**:45-52

[69] Bylund N, Hultcrantz M, Jonsson L, Marsk E. Quality of life in Bell's palsy: Correlation with Sunnybrook and

House-Brackmann over time. The Laryngoscope. 2021;**131**:E612-E618

[70] Wysocki J. Cadaveric dissections based on observations of injuries to the temporal bone structures following head trauma. Skull Base. 2005;**15**:99-106

[71] Ishman SL, Friedland DR. Temporal bone fractures: Traditional classification and clinical relevance. The Laryngoscope. 2004;**114**:1734-1741

[72] Antoniades E, Psillas G, Polyzoidis K, Patsalas I. Patient-assessed outcomes following temporal bone fractures. Diagnostics (Basel). 2022;**12**(2):547

[73] Gordts F, Foulon I, Hachimi-Idrissi S. Basilar skull fractures: The petrous bone. B-ENT. 2016;**12**(Suppl. 26):193-201

[74] Johnson F, Semaan MT, Megerian CA. Temporal bone fracture: Evaluation and management in the modern era. Otolaryngologic Clinics of North America. 2008;**41**:597-618

[75] Psillas G, Constantinidis J, Printza A, Vital V. Prognoseabschätzung der peripheren Fazialisparese: Ist der minimal-nerve-excitability-test noch zeitgemäss? [estimating the prognosis of peripheral facial paralysis: Is the minimal nerve excitability test still up to date?]. HNO. 2007;**55**:625-629

[76] Magliulo G, Ciniglio AM, Iannella G, Artico M. Petrous bone fractures violating otic capsule. Otology & Neurotology. 2012;**33**:1558-1561

[77] Voola M, Távora-Viera D. Quality of life handicap measured in patients with profound unilateral or bilateral deafness. Tasman Medical Journal. 2021;**3**:52-56

[78] Kurihara YY, Fujikawa A, Tachizawa N, Takaya M, Ikeda H, Starkey J. Temporal bone trauma: Typical CT and MRI appearances and important points for evaluation. Radiographics. 2020;**40**:1148-1162

[79] Hill-Feltham PR, Johansson ML, Hodgetts WE, Ostevik AV, McKinnon BJ, Monksfield P, et al. Hearing outcome measures for conductive and mixed hearing loss treatment in adults: A scoping review. International Journal of Audiology. 2021;**60**:239-245

[80] Roberts LE, Eggermont JJ, Caspary DM, Shore SE, Melcher JR, Kaltenbach JA. Ringing ears: The neuroscience of tinnitus. The Journal of Neuroscience. 2010;**30**:14972-14979

[81] Komiya H, Eggermont JJ. Spontaneous firing activity of cortical neurons in adult cats with reorganized tonotopic map following pure-tone trauma. Acta Oto-Laryngologica. 2000;**120**:750-756

[82] Fagelson MA. The association between tinnitus and posttraumatic stress disorder. American Journal of Audiology. 2007;**16**:107-117

[83] Singh G, Singh B, Singh D. Prospective study of 'otological injury secondary to head trauma'. Indian Journal of Otolaryngology - Head & Neck Surgery. 2013;**65**(Suppl. 3):498-504

[84] Livingston G, Sommerlad A, Orgeta V, Costafreda SG, Huntley J, Ames D, et al. Dementia prevention, intervention, and care. The Lancet (London, England). 2017;**390**:2673-2734

[85] Lin FR, Ferrucci L, An Y, Goh JO, Doshi J, Metter EJ, et al. Association of hearing impairment with brain volume changes in older adults. NeuroImage. 2014;**90**:84-92

[86] Rigters SC, Bos D, Metselaar M, Roshchupkin GV, Baatenburg de Jong RJ,

Ikram MA, et al. Hearing impairment is associated with smaller brain volume in aging. Frontiers in Aging Neuroscience. 2017;**9**:2

[87] Ray J, Popli G, Fell G. Association of cognition and age-related hearing impairment in the English longitudinal study of ageing. JAMA Otolaryngology. Head & Neck Surgery. 2018;**144**:876-882

[88] Assi H, Moore RD, Ellemberg D, et al. Sensitivity to sounds in sport-related concussed athletes: A new clinical presentation of hyperacusis. Scientific Reports. 2018;**8**:9921

[89] Lew HL, Jerger JF, Guillory SB, et al. Auditory dysfunction in traumatic brain injury. Journal of Rehabilitation Research and Development. 2007;**44**:921-928

[90] Kisilevski V, Podoshin L, Ben-David J, et al. Results of otovestibular tests in mild head injuries. The International Tinnitus Journal. 2001;**7**:118-121

[91] Attias J, Zwecker-Lazar I, Nageris B, et al. Dysfunction of the auditory efferent system in patients with traumatic brain inju- ries with tinnitus and hyperacusis. Journal of Basic and Clinical Physiology and Pharmacology. 2005;**16**:117-126

[92] Knoll R, Lubner RJ. Brodsky J auditory quality-of-life measures in patients with traumatic brain injury and normal pure tone audiometry. Otolaryngology and Head and Neck Surgery. 2020;**163**(6):1250-1254

[93] Zuccotti A, Kuhn S, Johnson SL, et al. Lack of brain-derived neurotrophic factor hampers inner hair cell synapse physiology, but protects against noise-induced hearing loss. The Journal of Neuroscience. 2012;**32**(25):8545-8553

[94] Lurie MHDH, Hawkins VE. Acoustic trauma of the organ of Corti in Guinea pigs. The Laryngoscope. 1944;**54**:375-386

[95] Lindquist SE, Schuknecht HF. Stimulation deafness: A study of hearing losses resulting from exposure to noise or to blast impulses. Journal of Comparative and Physiological Psychology. Oct 1954;**47**(5):406-411

[96] Zhou D, Xu W, He L. Histopathology of nonacoustic labyrinth following head injury in Guinea pigs. Zhonghua Er Bi Yan Hou Ke Za Zhi. 1994;**29**(6):350-352

[97] Bartholomew RA, Lubner RJ, Knoll RM, Ghanad I, Jung D, Nadol JB Jr, et al. Labyrinthine concussion: Historic otopathologic antecedents of a challenging diagnosis. Laryngoscope Investigative Otolaryngology. 2020;**5**(2):267-277

[98] Hoffer ME, Balaban C, Gottshall K, et al. Blast exposure: Vestibular consequences and associated characteristics. Otology & Neurotology. 2010;**31**:232-236

[99] Collins MW, Iverson GL, Lovell MR, et al. On-field predictors of neuropsychologyical and symptoms deficit following sports-related concussion. Clinical Journal of Sport Medicine. 2003;**13**:222-229

[100] Fife TD, Kalra D. Persistent vertigo and dizziness after mild traumatic brain injury. Annals of the New York Academy of Sciences. 2015;**1343**:97-105

[101] Miura M, Goto F, Inagaki Y, Nomura Y, Oshima T, Sugaya N. The effect of comorbidity between tinnitus and dizziness on perceived handicap, psychological distress, and quality of life. Frontiers in Neurology. 2017;**8**:722

[102] Smith PF, Horii A, Russell N, Bilkey DK, Zheng Y, Liu P, et al. The effects of vestibular lesions on hippocampal function in rats. Progress in Neurobiology. 2005;**75**(6):391-405

[103] Giummarra MJ, Gibson SJ, Georgiou-Karistianis N, Bradshaw JL. Mechanisms underlying embodiment, disembodiment and loss of embodiment. Neuroscience and Biobehavioral Reviews. 2008;**32**:143-160

[104] Lopez C, Lenggenhager B, Blanke O. How vestibular stimulation interacts with illusory hand ownership. Consciousness and Cognition. 2010;**19**(1):33-47

Chapter 4

Oropharyngeal Carcinomas: New Markers for their Diagnosis

Arushi Tomar, Sharon John and Shalini Gupta

Abstract

Oropharyngeal squamous cell carcinoma (OPSCC), the most common cancer of the head and neck, has increasing incident rates in some geographic locations, like Southeast Asia. This tumor, influenced by both epigenetic as well as environmental factors, such as tobacco as well as alcohol, requires management by controlling both the aforementioned factors. In order to control the epigenetic factors, the molecular changes that occur as a result of the genetic changes need to be identified beforehand so that personalized care can be provided to the patient. Therefore, a preliminary diagnosis of OSCC is necessary for prompt treatment, preventing increased morbidity. These markers are the end result of protein expression that may be seen either inside the cytoplasm or the nucleus. So, this present chapter highlights some molecular markers that may help in the diagnosis of these oropharyngeal carcinomas, which may help in providing an increased understanding of the molecular mechanism underlying the disease progression.

Keywords: oropharyngeal carcinoma, progression, molecular marker, mechanism, prognosis

1. Introduction

The most common type of cancer in the head and neck is called oropharyngeal squamous cell carcinoma (OPSCC). It is defined as cancer of the oropharynx, the middle part of the pharynx. It includes the tonsils, the base and posterior third of the tongue, the soft palate, and the posterior and lateral pharyngeal walls. OPSCC is on the rise in the modern world. OPSCC has been ranked as the sixth most common cancer worldwide, whereas in countries like India, it is the most common cancer among males, surpassing the number of lung cancer cases [1]. In females, it has been ranked after cervical and breast cancer, but still, the cases are seen increasing in number. This carries an even worse prognosis as compared to breast cancer. The risk factors for the development of oral cancers are multitude, which range from environmental exposures like sunlight to usage of tobacco products (smoked and smokeless) as well as alcohol to the induction of carcinogenesis by viruses [2].

One can distinguish between two types of oropharyngeal cancer: non-HPV-associated cancer, which is mostly caused by alcohol and tobacco use, and HPV-associated cancer, which is caused by an oral human papillomavirus infection. Nearly 90% of HPV-positive oropharyngeal malignancies are caused by HPV-16, and the frequency is higher in men than in women. The tonsils and base of the tongue had much greater rates of HPV-associated OPSCC. Younger people who smoke and drink less are more likely to be affected by HPV-associated OPSCC; a higher proportion of men and more oral sex partners are reported.

The oral mucosa is exposed to the HPV infection in HPV-associated OPSCC, which lingers and does not go away. A precancerous lesion that may or may not regress can result from this persistence. It will ultimately lead to invasive OPSCC if it does not. Within 10 years, persistent HPV infections may develop into aggressive malignancy. Most of these illnesses do, however, go away after a year or two.

The complicated process of carcinogenesis involves the activation of oncogenes and the silencing of tumor suppressor genes over a number of steps, genes, and stages. Therefore, understanding the molecular pathogenesis and protein formation underlying disease progression is as important for diagnosis as knowing the causative agent and genes. This knowledge would help to improve patient outcomes by not only understanding the disease process but also identifying and preventing the disease in advance [3]. Besides directly invading the tissues, oropharyngeal cancer has the ability to spread via lymphatic and blood vessels. The three main signs of oropharyngeal cancer are dysphagia, odynophagia, and sore throat. Based on the biopsy results of the afflicted tissue, a diagnosis is formed. Surgery, radiation, chemotherapy, or a mix of these treatments are used as forms of treatment.

The progression from mild and moderate dysplasia to severe dysplasia/carcinoma *in situ* is caused by the accumulation of genetic alterations in patients with oropharyngeal squamous cell carcinoma. However, the tumor begins deep within the tonsillar crypt epithelium in the majority of HPV-positive oropharyngeal malignancies. This explains why a superficial brush biopsy or visual inspection fails to detect certain tumors [4].

Depending on where the tumor is located, patients with oropharyngeal cancer may exhibit a wide range of symptoms. The most typical symptoms include otalgia, a lump in the neck, dysphagia, odynophagia, dysarthria, and a chronic sore throat. Patients may also report experiencing hematemesis, unexplained weight loss, and voice abnormalities (hoarseness). A physical examination of the oropharynx may reveal a red or white area on the tonsils, soft palate, posterior and lateral pharyngeal walls, or base or posterior third of the tongue, along with an ulcer. In addition to this, the other methods of evaluation include the combination of both invasive and noninvasive methods, which includes imaging such as magnetic resonance imaging (MRI), computed tomography (CT) scans, plain radiography, and ultrasonography. Invasive methods include the biopsy sample collected, which can undergo routine histopathological examination, and various molecular diagnostic methods, one of which is taken into consideration in this chapter, as mentioned below, is immunohistochemistry (IHC).

IHC is a potent laboratory technique that makes use of the particular binding between an antibody and antigen to identify and localize specific antigens in cells and tissue. The light microscope is most frequently used to detect and examine antigens in tissue samples. IHC is becoming a common tool in many domains used in research settings, and it is a crucial supplementary method for clinical diagnoses in anatomic pathology. It is a hybrid of immunology and histology that is employed in prognostication, therapy response prediction, and illness diagnosis. IHC is widely used to help classify neoplasms, identify the site of genesis of a metastatic tumor, and find small tumor cell foci that are not noticeable with standard hematoxylin and eosin (H&E) staining. The process, which is mostly applied to wax blocks with paraffin-embedded tissue embedded in them, involves first drying the tissue and then incubating it with antibodies that have been tagged with a fluorescent molecule. The fluorescence that is released after binding is then seen under a microscope. Positive reactions are typically observed as brown color, which can appear as granular staining or as a diffuse shape.

Antigen retrieval (AR), which entails pre-treating tissue to recover antigens obscured by fixation and increase their accessibility to antibody binding, is typically the first stage in immunohistochemistry (IHC). This method, which Shi et al. originally reported, has considerably raised IHC's sensitivity and, as a result, tremendously broadened its use. Depending on the particular target antigen and antibody, there are a number of different ways to retrieve antigens; nevertheless, the majority of them entail chemically or physically rupturing protein cross-links created by fixation, like formalin. While chemical procedures include denaturant treatment and enzyme digestion, many physical treatments—such as heat and ultrasound—also combine the two. One such example is the combination of chemical and heat therapy. The most widely used technique at the moment is microwave oven-based heat-induced antigen retrieval (HIAR).

In order to maximize contrast between positively stained tissue and nonspecific background staining, the primary antibody—which can be monoclonal or polyclonal—is titrated at the highest primary antibody dilution possible to avoid waste. Tests are conducted on a series of tissues with the appropriate positive control using dilutions that are more and less concentrated than the stated dilution. Typically, the dilution recommended by the manufacturer or documented in the literature for the target tissue is the first one examined. To achieve the best staining, this can be used with different secondary antibody dilution combinations depending on the specific AR technique and chromogen. An antibody concentration of 1–5 μg/mL is often advised for the first titration.

Either the primary antibody or the secondary antibody that is directed against the immunoglobulin of the animal that produced the primary antibody needs to be labeled in order to see the antigen-antibody interaction under light microscopy. The direct method requires the primary antibody to be labeled and applied to the tissue in a single, fast step. Nevertheless, because there is no signal amplification, a higher antibody concentration is needed, and each primary antibody must be labeled, making this method uncommon. By labeling the secondary antibody in the indirect technique, signal amplification and versatility with various primary antibodies are made possible. Many labels can be used, such as fluorescent substances and enzymes that, when incubated with a chromogenic substrate like diaminobenzidine (DAB), yield a colored result, such as horseradish peroxidase or alkaline phosphatase. Fluorescence chemicals can also be used in immunofluorescence procedures; however, these methods need a fluorescence microscope. Due to endogenous biotin binding, the avidin-biotin-peroxidase approach has strong background staining and is now mostly out of use. A dextran polymer backbone is coupled to many peroxidase molecules and secondary antibodies in polymer-based techniques, which enhance sensitivity.

Background staining may result from endogenous peroxidase activity or nonspecific antibody binding, which is more common in polyclonal antibodies and more problematic in tissues like bone marrow that have a high concentration of hematopoietic components. Preincubation using normal serum from the same species as the secondary antibody or with a commercially available universal blocking agent can reduce nonspecific antibody binding. Before applying the antibody, the tissue can be pre-treated with hydrogen peroxide-containing solutions to reduce endogenous enzyme activity.

Every run should include both positive and negative quality control. Quality control is vital. To ensure that the control tissue experiences the same reaction circumstances as the sample tissue, positive controls should ideally be run on the same slide as the tissue of interest. Positive controls are tissues that contain an antigen that is known to stain with a particular antibody. Negative controls are samples of tissue stained under the same conditions without the primary antibody or with a non-immune immunoglobulin from the same species in order to rule out the possibility of nonspecific antibody interaction with the secondary antibody. False positives and negatives can result from a variety of circumstances, including preparation and fixation, in addition to the immunohistochemistry approach itself.

The markers that have been described in the following chapter includes AJUBA, S-100, GLUT-1, and NESTIN, which have been studied by the authors by using the cases retrieved from the archives and expression noted in different grades of oropharyngeal carcinoma. Therefore, the present chapter focuses in the subsequent sections on the details of the mechanism of action of the markers and their expression, indicating their diagnostic as well as prognostic significance.

2. Mechanism of function of AJUBA protein

LIM-protein A member of the Zyxin/AJUBA family is AJUBA. The AJUBA protein family functions as a negative regulator of the Hippo pathway, which can restrict the growth of tissues and the proliferation of cells. It oscillates between cytoplasm as well as nucleus depending on the exporting sequence in the Pre-LIM domain along with the localization sequence in the LIM domain. Tumor epithelial-mesenchymal transition (EMT), migration, metastasis, and patient survival are under the purview of AJUBA [5]. Allows transcription corepressor and alpha-catenin binding activity, involved in a number of functions, such as the control of the cellular response to hypoxia, the positive control of miRNA-mediated gene silencing, and the negative regulation of hippocampal signaling. Functions either before or after miRNA-mediated gene silencing, as well as positively regulating the formation of protein-containing complexes.

3. Association of AJUBA protein with cases of OPSCC

This protein is seen to be expressed inside during the proliferation of cells, which is a factor responsible not only for dysplastic activity but also for tumorigenesis. This was observed to be regulating the nuclear activity inside the cells, and no activity was seen inside the cytoplasm of the cells in cases of oropharyngeal carcinoma. The differentiated cell, even after they have metastasized to the connective tissue, showed negative expression in cases of carcinomas, whereas this protein has been found to indicate the proliferative potential of the cell but cannot be seen in cells that have undergone differentiation, metaplastic or anaplastic changes. Therefore, this can help in identifying only the well-differentiated cases of oropharyngeal carcinomas but not the cases of moderately poorly differentiated carcinomas (**Figure 1**).

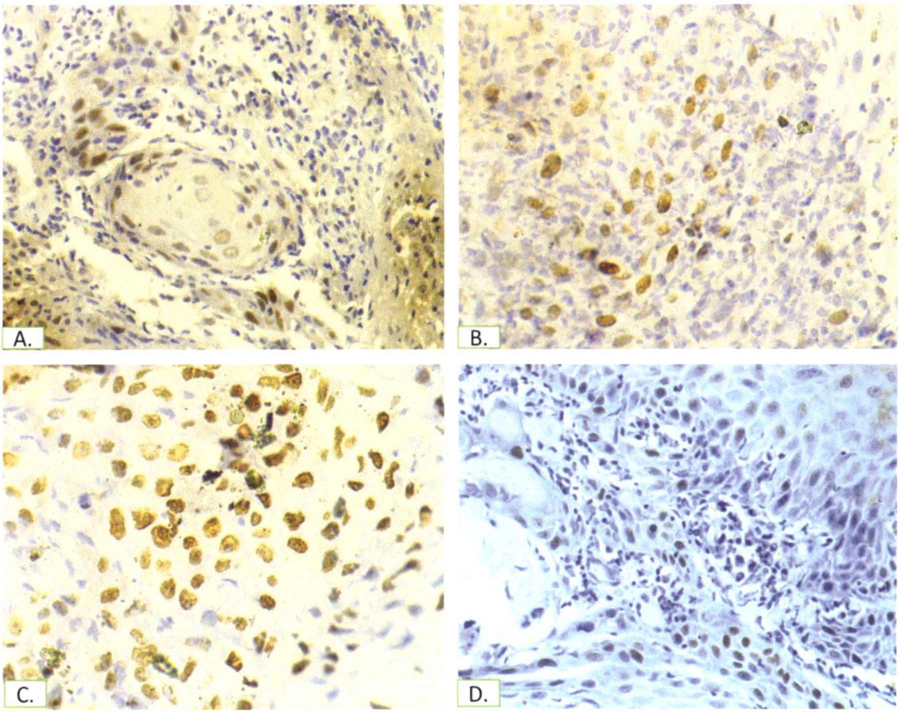

Figure 1.
Positive expression of AJUBA in well-differentiated OPSCC.

4. Mechanism of function of S100 protein

Low-molecular weight calcium-binding proteins (9–14 kDa) in the S100 subfamily are diverse and exhibit both structural and functional variation. It functions extracellularly, intracellularly, or both and is necessary for both inflammation and cellular homeostasis. In a healthy cell, S100 members are involved in many different processes, such as the storage and transfer of calcium (calcium homeostasis). Alarmins (DAMPs), antimicrobial peptides, pro-inflammatory stimulators, chemo-attractants, and metal scavengers are among the S100 isoforms that have been demonstrated to have significant functions in the immune system during an innate immune response. S100B, S100A1, S1 00A8 (nitrosylation), S100A8/A9, S100A11 (phosphorylation), S100A8/A9 (carboxymethylation), S100A3 (citrullination), S100A11 (transamination), S100A14 (myristoylation), S100A1 (glutathionylation), S100A8/A9 (oxidation), and S100A4 (sumoylation) are notable examples of the extensive post-translational modifications that S100 protein members go through in order to gain functional activity [6].

S100 protein profiles are characteristic of cancers and can be subtype- and stage-specific. While S100A8 and S100A9 expression positively correlates with mesenchymal subtypes in gliomas, S100B expression positively correlates with proneuronal, neuronal, and classic subtypes but not with mesenchymal subtypes. Comprehensive investigations of S100 protein expression have not been conducted, despite the availability of protein signatures from colorectal, melanoma, prostate, breast, and head and neck malignancies. However, comparing the S100 protein expression levels in human malignancies reveals both clear trends and noteworthy deviations. Most malignancies exhibit several S100 family members' dysregulation, which usually includes upregulation. S100P, one family member, is elevated in every cancer that has been studied, while the other S100 family members are upregulated in the majority of cancers, but not all of them are cancers. Head and neck malignancies and ocular tumors are the two exceptions, where 11 out of 13 and 6 out of 12 dysregulated S100 proteins, respectively, are downregulated. Some family members' conflicting expression profiles have been described; these could be related to cellular distribution, illness stage, cancer subtype, or problems with S100 protein and/or mRNA detection. S100 protein expression patterns can help with prognosis and/or diagnosis, provide information on available treatments, and track a patient's response to therapy [7, 8].

5. Association of S100 protein with cases of OPSCC

Through interactions with a variety of target proteins, including enzymes, cytoskeletal subunits, receptors, transcription factors, and nucleic acids, S100 proteins have been implicated in the regulation of proliferation, differentiation, apoptosis, Ca2+ homeostasis, energy metabolism, inflammation, and migration/invasion. This family has been found to be downregulated in various types of cancers and acts as a specific marker for neural cells, myofibroblasts, and other mesenchymal cells. Therefore, the expression of this protein was seen in cases with a worse prognosis, that is, in cases of poorly-differentiated oropharyngeal carcinomas, where neural invasion was seen. Also, the expression of this protein was also noted in proliferating cells inside the nucleus but not inside the cytoplasm. Therefore, in the connective tissue, the expression was not noted in epithelial cells, but in well-differentiated tumors, it was noted inside the epithelial cells. Therefore, similar to AJUBA, S100 can be used for diagnosing proliferating status but not the differentiated or the metaplasia/anaplasia associated with the tumors (**Figure 2**).

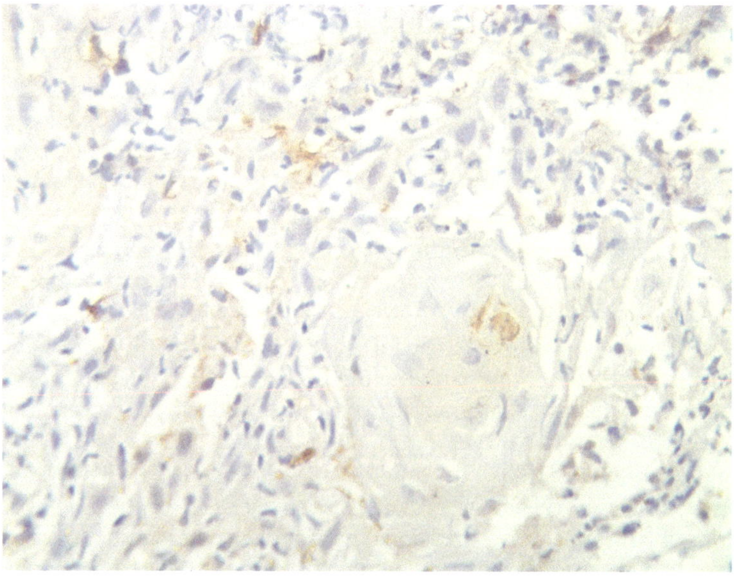

Figure 2.
Positive expression of S-100 in well-differentiated OPSCC.

6. Mechanism of function of GLUT1 protein

Glucose transporters (GLUTs) assist in the intracellular transportation of glucose, a primary source of energy for all cells. There are two different kinds of these transporters: facilitative GLUTs and sodium-dependent GLUTs. They have substrate specificity and are distributed in a way distinct from a given tissue. GLUT1 (facilitative GLUT) is one of these transporters that is widely distributed throughout the body's tissues and aids in the basal absorption of glucose. Since an embryo's implantation, GLUT1 has been known to perform a variety of physiological tasks in the body. It has also been linked to diseases, such as malignancies. The glucose transporter 1 (GLUT1) protein facilitates the transport of glucose across membranes by switching between two conformations: outward-open (OOP) and inward-open (IOP). This protein facilitates the passive transport of glucose down a concentration gradient. It consists of 12 hydrophobic transmembrane α-helices with a glycosylated extracellular loop sandwiched between transmembrane helices 1 and 2, and both N and C terminals on the cytoplasmic side. Maximum expression levels in proliferating cells' plasma membranes during an embryo's early development. High concentrations of it are found in the brain, skeletal muscle, and myocardium during the postnatal period of nursing. From this time onward into adulthood, the expression of GLUT1 decreases with the exception of the brain, and the amount of tissue-specific isoforms increases [9, 10].

7. Association of GLUT1 protein with cases of OPSCC

In OPSCC, increased expression of GLUT1 is found to be associated with increased aggressiveness of tumor, also it can help in determining patient overall survival as well as prognosis. Due to the fact that increased metabolism occurs in cells that are in a more proliferative stage, therefore expression of this category of protein can be inside the nucleus of the cells. Thus, it can be seen to be expressed in more proliferating cells as well as the cells undergoing differentiation. Glycogen content is always inversely connected with GLUT-1 expression in both pre-neoplastic lesions and normal mucosa; cells with varying degrees of dysplasia associated with elevated GLUT-1 expression show lower glycogen storage and intense glycogen accumulation in normal mucosa. Such expression of GLUT-1 is also found to be inversely correlated with the extension of the proliferating compartment, showing an association between glycogen storage and tumor cell differentiation in SCC. Therefore, as seen in the abovementioned proteins, this marker is also seen in well-differentiated cases of oropharyngeal carcinoma and can also act as a prognostic marker for the cases as such.

8. Mechanism of function of NESTIN protein

The NES gene in humans' codes for the protein NESTIN. Type VI intermediate filament (IF) protein is called NESTIN, an acronym for neuroepithelial stem cell protein. The majority of these intermediate filament proteins' expression occurs in nerve cells, where they are thought to be involved in the axon's radial growth. The DMN gene has seven transcripts: desmuslin/synemin β and synemin α in muscle cells, syncoilin (also in muscle cells), NESTIN and α-internexin in nerve cells, and desmuslin/synemin β and heavy (NF-H), medium (NF-M), and light neurofilament

(NF-L) proteins. In tissues, most members of this category preferentially coassemble as heteropolymers. Of all the IF proteins, NESTIN has the longest tail domain (C-terminus) and the shortest head domain (N-terminus) structurally. The molecular weight of NESTIN is high (240 kDa) [11].

Many different types of cells express NESTIN during development; however, this expression is typically fleeting and does not continue into adulthood. Neural precursor cells in the subgranular zone are one adult organism where NESTIN is expressed, and this may be the instance for which NESTIN is most well-known. In the early phases of development, NESTIN, an intermediate filament protein, is expressed in proliferating cells in the peripheral and central nervous systems, as well as in myogenic and other tissues. Tissue-specific intermediate filament proteins replace downregulated NESTIN during differentiation. NESTIN is substituted by cell type-specific intermediate filaments, such as neurofilaments and glial fibrillary acidic protein (GFAP), during neuro- and gliogenesis. In pathological circumstances, such as the development of a glial scar following damage to the central nervous system or during the regeneration of damaged muscle tissue, NESTIN expression is reinduced in adults [12].

9. Association of NESTIN protein with cases of OPSCC

Follicle stem cells and their immediate, differentiated progeny exhibit NESTIN, a protein marker specific to neural stem cells. A plentiful and convenient source of pluripotent adult stem cells that are actively proliferating is the area around the hair follicle bulge. Hair follicle stem cells are marked by green fluorescent protein (GFP), whose expression is regulated by the NESTIN regulatory element in transgenic mice. *In vitro*, these cells can develop into smooth muscle cells, neurons, glia, keratinocytes, and melanocytes. For the treatment of peripheral nerve damage, hair follicle stem cells offer an efficient, readily available, autologous source of stem cell [13].

NESTIN's expression and distribution in mitotically active cells indicate that it regulates the formation and disassembly of intermediate filaments, which are involved in cell remodeling alongside other structural proteins. NESTIN's function in dynamic cells, specifically the structural organization of the cell, seems to be carefully regulated by phosphorylation. This is especially true of its integration with vimentin or α-internexin into heterogeneous intermediate filaments. Furthermore, due to data showing a link between NESTIN expression and this cell type *in vivo*, NESTIN expression has been widely employed as a marker for progenitor cells of the central nervous system in several circumstances. As a result, this serves as a marker for angiogenesis and may be used to anticipate the advancement of different phases of abnormal cell proliferation [14].

10. Conclusion

Oral as well as oropharyngeal carcinoma is now seen on toward an increasing trend across the world, most commonly seen in developing countries as a result of the increased trend toward the use of tobacco concomitant with alcohol. The tumor can be categorized on the basis of differentiating potential of the epithelial cells as well as the invasion of the epithelial cells into the connective tissue. The more the proliferating potential of the cells, the more differentiated a tumor can be, which is associated with increased patient outcomes as well as prognosis. The proliferating potential of the cells can, therefore be confirmed by the expression of the abovementioned proteins that can help in determining the course of action of the tumors, thereby providing patient-centered approach for decreasing the mortality and morbidity of the tumors as such.

Author's contribution

All the authors contributed equally.

Author details

Arushi Tomar*, Sharon John and Shalini Gupta
Department of Oral Pathology and Microbiology, King George's Medical University, Lucknow, India

*Address all correspondence to: arushitomar704@gmail.com

References

[1] Nokovitch L, Maquet C, Crampon F, Taihi I, Roussel LM, Obongo R, et al. Oral cavity squamous cell carcinoma risk factors: State of the art. Journal of Clinical Medicine. 2023;**12**(9):3264

[2] Ferlay J, Colombet M, Soerjomataram I, Mathers C, Parkin DM, Piñeros M, et al. Estimating the global cancer incidence and mortality in 2018: GLOBOCAN sources and methods. International Journal of Cancer. 2019;**144**:1941-1953

[3] WHO Classification of Tumours Editorial Board. Head and Neck Tumours. 5th ed. Lyon: IARC; 2023

[4] Wood HM, Daly C, Chalkley R, et al. The genomic road to invasion examining the similarities and differences in the genomes of associated oral pre-cancer and cancer samples. Genome Medicine. 2017;**9**:53

[5] Jia H, Peng H, Hou Z. Ajuba: An emerging signal transducer in oncogenesis. Pharmacological Research. 2020;**151**:104546

[6] Liang XH, Zhang GX, Zeng YB, Yang HF, Li WH, Liu QL, et al. LIM protein JUB promotes epithelial-mesenchymal transition in colorectal cancer. Cancer Science. 2014;**105**(6):660-666

[7] Hermann A, Donato R, Weiger TM, Chazin WJ. S100 calcium binding proteins and ion channels. Frontiers in Pharmacology. 2012;**3**:67

[8] Marenholz I, Heizmann CW, Fritz G. S100 proteins in mouse and man: From evolution to function and pathology (including an update of the nomenclature). Biochemical and Biophysical Research Communications. 2004;**322**:1111-1122

[9] Ohba S, Fujii H, Ito S, Fujimaki M, Matsumoto F, Furukawa M, et al. Overexpression of GLUT-1 in the invasion front is associated with depth of oral squamous cell carcinoma and prognosis. Journal of Oral Pathology & Medicine. 2010;**39**:74-78

[10] Oliver RJ, Woodwards RT, Sloan P, Thakker NS, Stratford IJ, Airley RE. Prognostic value of facilitative glucose transporter Glut-1 in oral squamous cell carcinomas treated by surgical resection; results of EORTC translational research fund studies. European Journal of Cancer. 2004;**40**:503-507

[11] Bernal A, Arranz L. Nestin-expressing progenitor cells: Function, identity and therapeutic implications. Cellular and Molecular Life Sciences. 2018 Jun;**75**(12):2177-2195

[12] Carlsson L, Li Z, Paulin D, Thornell LE. Nestin is expressed during development and in myotendinous and neuromuscular junctions in wild type and desmin knock-out mice. Experimental Cell Research. 1999;**251**:213-223

[13] Wiese C, Rolletschek A, Kania G, Blyszczuk P, Tarasov KV, et al. Nestin expression - a property of multi-lineage progenitor cells? Cellular and Molecular Life Sciences. 2004;**61**:2510-2522

[14] Michalczyk K, Ziman M. Nestin structure and predicted function in cellular cytoskeletal organisation. Histology and Histopathology. 2005;**20**:665-671

Chapter 5

Pathogenetic Action of Viruses in Head and Neck Cancer

Eleni Litsou

Abstract

Head and neck cancer (HNC) represents a heterogeneous group of neoplasms with different biological and clinical behavior, which develops in the upper parts of the respiratory and digestive tract outside the esophagus. The majority (>90%) of HNCs arise from squamous epithelium and are classified as head and neck squamous cell carcinomas (HNSCCs). The main anatomical localizations of HNSCCs concern the paranasal sinuses, oral cavity, salivary glands, larynx, pharynx, and nasal cavity. Oncogenic viruses play an important role in the development of HNC. Human papillomavirus (HPV) has been extensively studied in relation to oropharyngeal carcinoma, but other oncogenic viruses also contribute to the HNC onset. This chapter summarizes advances in the pathogenesis, epidemiology and detection of oncogenic viruses implicated in HNC, recognizing the established role of HPV and discussing its relationship with other viruses. Epstein-Barr virus in particular has been associated with lymphoma and nasopharyngeal carcinoma. Merkel cell polyomavirus has been associated with a subset of HNC and human herpesvirus 8 is linked to Kaposi sarcoma. Hepatitis viruses have also been investigated for possible association with HNC.

Keywords: head and neck cancer, oncogenic viruses, human papillomavirus, Epstein-Barr virus, human herpesvirus 8, Merkel cell polyomavirus, hepatitis B, hepatitis C

1. Introduction

Head and neck cancer (HNC) represents a heterogeneous group of neoplasms with different biological and clinical behavior, which develops in the upper parts of the digestive and respiratory tract, outside the esophagus, including regions such as the salivary glands, nasal cavity, oral cavity, paranasal sinuses, larynx and pharynx.

Thyroid cancer, skin cancer affecting the head and neck, and ear cancer are often managed separately from traditional HNC despite their anatomical location in this region. In addition, lymphomas are also not traditionally classified as HNCs but may involve the head and neck region [1]. Approximately 90% of HNCs are squamous cell carcinomas [2].

Head and neck squamous cell carcinoma (HNSCC) is the 6th most common neoplasm worldwide, representing 3% of all neoplasms, with over 600,000 new cases and 350,000 deaths annually [3]. About 5% of HNC is made up of melanoma, lymphoma and sarcoma. In children, primary malignant tumors of the head and neck constitute approximately 5% of all malignant tumors affecting them. The most common tumors

IntechOpen

of the head and neck in children are lymphoma and rhabdomyosarcoma and the most commonly affected areas are the cervix (70%) and the nasopharynx and oropharynx (16%) [4]. With the exception of salivary gland cancer, men are affected more often than women in a ratio of 3:1, reaching 8:1 in the case of laryngeal cancer.

Because of its complex genesis, heterogeneous character and variable response to treatment, HNC presents substantial hurdles for therapeutic management [5]. HNC remains a global burden and highlights the need for a better understanding of the underlying mechanisms.

Among the multifaceted factors in the development of HNC, oncogenic viruses have appeared as an important factor profoundly influencing both the starting and progression of these malignant tumors [6]. These encompass the full spectrum of virology and include both large double-stranded DNA viruses (like Epstein-Barr virus (EBV) and Kaposi's sarcoma herpesvirus (KSHV; also known as human herpesvirus 8 (HHV8)) and small double-stranded DNA viruses (like HPV and Merkel cell polyomavirus (MCV)), as well as complex exogenous retroviruses (like HTLV-I), positive-stranded RNA viruses (like hepatitis C virus (HCV) and DNA viruses with retroviral characteristics (like hepatitis B virus (HBV)). A clear molecular rule that definitively identifies or rules out an agent as a possible human tumor virus *a priori* does not exist. Furthermore, nearly every tumor virus has close cousins that do not cause cancer in humans. This suggests that while nearly all viruses have the capacity to cause cancer, only a very tiny percentage of them do so [7]. Seven human carcinogenic viruses are currently known as viruses with potential oncogenic dynamic in the head and neck region, including five DNA viruses: hepatitis B virus (HBV), Kaposi's sarcoma herpes virus or human herpes virus 8 (KSHV or HHV-8), Merkel cell polyomavirus (MCPV), Epstein-Barr virus (EBV) and human papillomavirus (HPV). There are also two RNA viruses, human T lymphotropic virus type 1 (HTLV-1) and hepatitis C virus (HCV). HTLV-1 is mainly associated with T-cell malignancies such as adult T-cell leukemia/lymphoma and HTLV-1-associated myelopathy/tropical spastic paraplegia, and rarely has direct involvement in HNC (**Table 1**) [8].

Virus	Genome type	Associated cancers in head and neck region
Human papillomavirus (HPV)	DNA	Oropharyngeal, laryngeal, oral cavity
Epstein-Barr virus (EBV)	DNA	Nasopharyngeal, Burkitt & Hodgkin lymphomas
Human herpesvirus 8 (HHV-8)	DNA	Kaposi's sarcoma, primary effusion lymphoma, multicentric Castleman disease, laryngeal
Merkel cell polyomavirus (MCPV)	DNA	Merkel cell carcinoma, head and neck squamous cell, oral squamous cell carcinomas
Hepatitis B virus (HBV)	DMA	Head and neck squamous cell carcinoma
Hepatitis C virus (HCV)	RNA	Head and neck squamous cell carcinoma, oral cavity
Human herpesvirus 1 (HHV-1)	DNA	Correlation with lip, oral cavity and pharynx
Cytomegalovirus (CMV)	DNA	Pro-oncogenic link with nasopharyngeal, protective effect with tumors of the lip/oral region and salivary glands
Human herpesviruses 2, 3, 6, 7 (HHV-2, HHV-3, HHV-6 and HHV-7)	DNA	Potential tumorigenic properties—not fully elucidated

Table 1.
HNCs-associated oncogenic viruses [8].

By interfering with the regulation of the cell cycle, evading immune monitoring and encouraging genomic instability, these viruses thwart cell transformation [9]. The early oncogenes E6 and E7, for instance, are overexpressed when HPV DNA is incorporated into host cells, inactivating the tumor suppressor proteins p53 and Rb, respectively [10]. About 70% of oropharyngeal malignancies (OPCs) in the US are caused by HPV, and the incidence of HPV-associated HNCs, particularly oropharyngeal squamous cell carcinoma (OPSCC), is rising sharply. This has a big effect on patient outcomes and clinical care [11]. In the same way, EBV is involved in almost all nasopharyngeal cancers and a considerable percentage of head and neck lymphomas, exhibiting complicated viral interactions in the tumor microenvironment [12].

Different HNC subtypes have distinct molecular fingerprints and viral profiles that indicate different biological activities and treatment responses [13]. Understanding how oncogenic viruses and host factors interact is essential for creating tailored treatment plans that effectively stop the progression of HNC while lowering treatment-associated morbidity. The identification and characterization of viral involvement in HNC has been transformed by advancements in detection techniques, including next-generation sequencing (NGS) [14], highly sensitive polymerase chain reaction (PCR) assays, and sophisticated imaging [15]. These methods improve patient outcomes by facilitating earlier diagnosis, improved prognosis and tailored treatment approximations.

This chapter's goal is to give a thorough review of the part oncogenic viruses play in HNC, with an emphasis on how they affect the onset and course of the disease. The goal is to clarify the various roles that HPV, EBV and other associated viruses play in various HNC subtypes by combining the most recent research on these viruses. In order to steer future research directions and improve diagnostic techniques in this difficult disease environment, it is imperative to comprehend the intricate connection between oncogenic viruses and HNCs.

2. Carcinogenesis

2.1 Process and stages of carcinogenesis

Carcinogenic transformation can be understood as the end result of a series of changes at the cellular level (**Figure 1**) [16] that lead to the loss of the control mechanisms of cell proliferation, differentiation and localization. It is a multistep process that often begins with exposure of the organism to carcinogenic agents (such as chemical carcinogens, radiation and viruses) and results in the creation of cells that have a proliferative and survival advantage through the induction of alterations in molecular pathways.

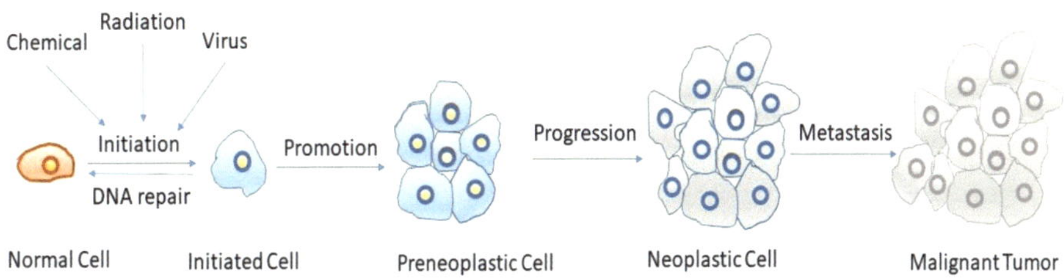

Figure 1.
Multistep process involved in carcinogenesis that transforms a normal cell into a malignant tumor [16].

Although in the case of some cancers, these molecular pathways have been determined, in most tumors, they remain unknown. In order for cancer to end up in the malignant phenotype, additional factors must act and cause additional genetic and epigenetic alterations, such as activation of oncogenes and deactivation of tumor suppressor genes [17]. In most cases of cancer, it remains unclear exactly which of the genetic changes causes the initiation of neoplasia, as well as what is the exact sequence of changes that ultimately lead to the cancerous phenotype [18].

These changes do not occur simultaneously, but, according to the theory of the multistage origin of cancer, accumulate over time, so that each mutation results in the creation of a large number of cells that act as a substrate for subsequent mutations [19]. In a seminal publication in 2000, Hanahan and Weinberg described six hallmarks of cancer: (a) acquisition of competence in proliferative signals, (b) unresponsiveness to signals that inhibit cell proliferation (tumor suppressor genes), (c) avoidance of apoptosis, (d) cell immortalization, (e) adequate angiogenesis and (f) infiltration and metastasis (**Figure 2**) [20].

Negrini et al. proposed the addition of genomic instability to these traits [21].

Cells can follow a wide range of routes before developing into cancerous tissue. Only a small percentage of tumors that are otherwise histologically identical may have mutations in certain target genes, such as ras or p53, within a given cancer type. Furthermore, early in some tumor growth pathways and late in others, mutations in specific oncogenes and tumor suppressor genes may arise. As a result, during these diverse progressions, the development of biological traits including resistance to apoptosis, prolonged angiogenesis and limitless replicative capacity may manifest at different times. As a result, there can be significant variation in the specific order in which skills are gained, both within and between tumors of the same kind (**Figure 3**). Additionally, a particular genetic event may help acquire multiple distinct capacities at the same time in some tumors, whereas in others, it may only partially contribute

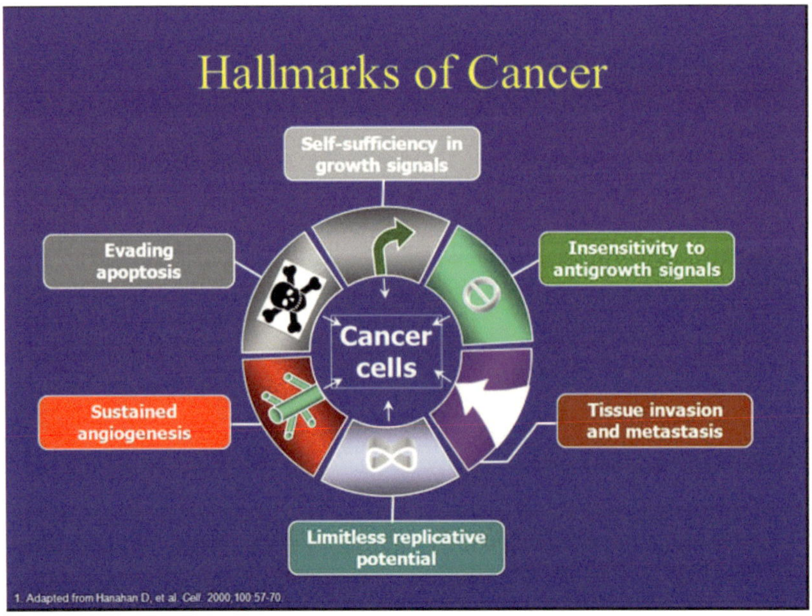

Figure 2.
Acquired capabilities of cancer [20].

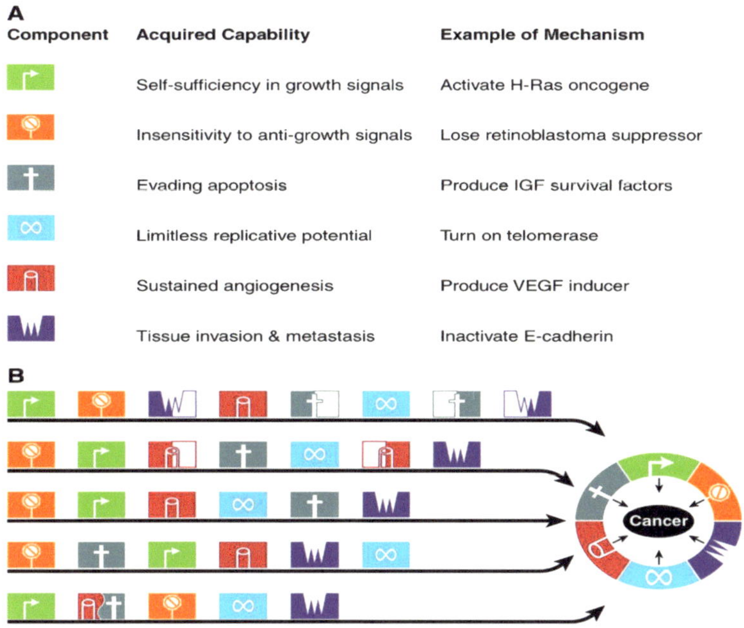

Figure 3.
Parallel pathways of tumorigenesis [20].

to the acquisition of a single skill. However, we think that the biological endpoints that are eventually reached—the characteristics that define cancer—will turn out to be the same for all tumor types, regardless of the order of the stages in these genetic pathways [20].

Cancer induction experiments in murine squamous skin epithelia have yielded models of carcinogenesis and three stages (**Figure 4**) of carcinogenesis have been proposed, which often overlap [22].

During the initiation stage, the genetic material of the cell is damaged by some endogenous or exogenous factor. If the damage is not repaired, it can lead to an irreversible mutation. In the promotion stage, further changes in the mutant cells are

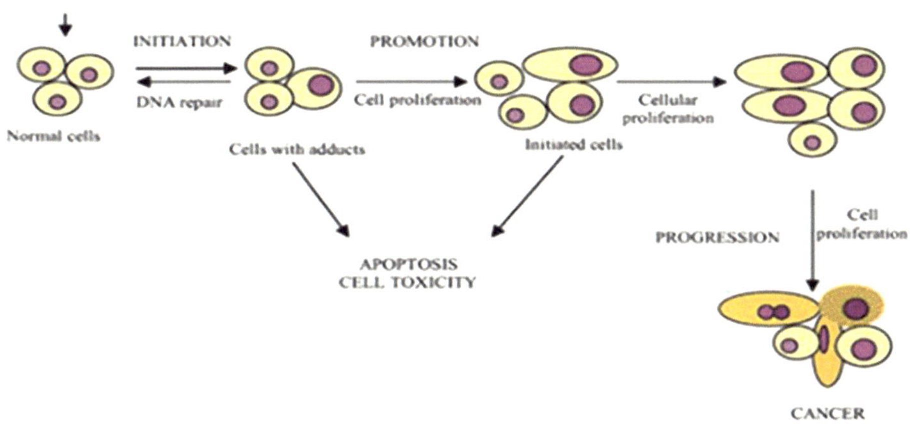

Figure 4.
The multistep nature of cancer development [22].

observed through epigenetic and no longer genetic mechanisms. The changes here concern the level of gene expression and include regulation of the transcription of genes responsible for cell growth, apoptosis and differentiation. Cells with altered gene expression and enzyme activity lead to altered clones. Phenotypically, this phase is manifested by the development of benign tumors. Finally, during the progression stage, additional genetic events occur, such as aneuploidy and loss of heterozygosity, which lead to cellular dysplasia, local infiltration of cancer cells and metastasis.

2.2 Models of carcinogenesis in the head and neck

The most popular theories for the development of squamous cell carcinoma in the head and neck are the multistep carcinogenesis and the field cancerization theory.

2.2.1 Multistep carcinogenesis

This is a theory based on the opinion that a series of successive events-steps lead to the development of invasive cancer. According to her HNC is created by a clone of cells that gradually accumulates many genetic and phenotypic lesions through a sequence of multiple steps (**Figure 4**) [22]. The first step, "initiation," is the interaction of a carcinogen with DNA to produce a permanent change in the genome. Initiation is a relatively random event. The second step, "promotion", takes place as the clone of cells undergoing the first step grows and proliferates to give an entire population of similar cells. This step is characterized by the development of precancerous lesions, eg oral or laryngeal leukoplakia. The third step, "progression", is the development of invasive cancer.

A direct indication of the correctness of this theory is a number of cytogenetic studies and especially studies of the change in the amount of DNA, aneuploidy, which highlight accumulations of non-random chromosomal changes in malignant lesions and a gradual increase in grade as the lesion develops into invasive cancer. Furthermore, this theory is supported by the measurements of cell proliferation indicators such as the intranuclear peptide PCNA (proliferating cell nuclear antigen) which seems to increase gradually and depending on the histological evolution of the damage.

2.2.2 Field cancerization

The principle of this theory is the view that respiratory and digestive malignancies do not develop in isolation but are the first focus in a wider field with increased risk [23]. The theory was formulated in 1953 by Slaughter [24] who, examining the epithelium from a large number of tissue sections from patients with squamous epithelial cancer of the oral cavity, pharynx and lips, found that very often close to the invasive cancer there was significant epithelial hyperplasia and dysplasia, while at least one other focus of cancer *in situ* was detected in tumors larger than 1 centimeter.

In the same study by Slaughter, multiple independent tumors were found in 11.9% of patients. So it was concluded that a large area of the mucosa had been irreversibly exposed to a carcinogen so that the development of cancer was inevitable.

The theory of field carcinogenesis also explains why, in oral cancer, even after successful treatment (e.g., complete surgical removal), a large percentage of second primary lesions with an unfavorable prognosis appear. According to the theory of field carcinogenesis, an entire epithelial area (field) subjected to long-term exposure to carcinogens is predisposed to the development of multiple cancerous foci, as well as precancerous lesions. The similarity between the gene profiles of carcinomas and their surrounding tissues has led to the hypothesis that the existence of such fields precedes the development of invasive carcinomas [25, 26]. There is evidence that these precancerous areas are preceded by a mutation in the p53 gene [25].

It has also been found that tumors that develop in such a background are clonally related to each other and derive from a common ancestor [27]. According to the hypothesis of clonal expansion, genetically altered epithelial cells of the basal layer begin to grow in a horizontal direction, along the basal and parabasal layers, forming at first a focus (patch) and later expanding into a field, which will eventually mutate focally into cancer [27, 28].

It has been shown that in at least 35% of oral and nasopharyngeal tumors, the tumor is surrounded by apparently normal but histologically altered epithelium. The clinical significance of this observation lies in the presence of genetically altered epithelium at the surgical margins of resected tumors in 70% of patients with HNSCCs, which means that, despite the surgical removal of the tumor, dysplastic epithelium remains in the patient and may in the future give genesis in relapses or in the development of a second primary focus [27]. The multifocality of these cancers is an important failure factor often observed in the treatment of oral cancer and has led to the development of chemoprevention, which is based on the administration of systemic therapy to protect the epithelium of the entire upper respiratory and digestive tract from follow the steps of stepwise carcinogenesis [26, 29].

3. Viral carcinogenesis

3.1 Introduction

Factors that can cause damage to genetic material, change cell metabolism and participate in neoplastic transformation include viruses. Viruses have played an important role in turning cancer research into the science of genetics. Much of what we know today about the mechanisms of oncogenetics comes from studies on viruses.

In conclusion, throughout the past 25–30 years, oncogenes have been important in the study of cancer both as possible human carcinogens and as instruments for the identification and investigation of cell signaling and cell growth control. RNA viruses seem prominent in the first stage of the effort, while DNA viruses are involved in both.

The recognition of the viral etiology of head and neck cancer and the clarification of the pathogenic oncogenic action of various viruses is also the purpose of this chapter.

3.2 Action's mechanisms of oncogenic viruses

Direct carcinogens, which express viral oncogenes that directly contribute to the transformation of cancer cells and indirect carcinogens, which most likely cause cancer through chronic infection and inflammation that ultimately results in carcinogenic mutations in host cells, are the two main categories into which infectious cancer agents, including viruses, have been separated [30, 31]. As is the case with malignancies linked to HPV, MCV, EBV and KSHV, each cancer cell by definition has a direct viral carcinogen that expresses at least one transcript to preserve the altered tumor cell phenotype [32–38]. Viruses are infectious agents that, in order to multiply, depend on the metabolic mechanism of their host cell, that is, they are obligate intracellular parasites.

The way viruses cause damage to the host cell varies. Some viruses inhibit the host cell's DNA, RNA or protein synthesis while retaining this ability for their own metabolism. Other viruses insert their own proteins into the cell membrane of the host cell and thereby affect its integrity. Many viruses multiply to large numbers inside the host cell and eventually cause lysis of the cell.

Finally, some viruses, by interfering with the metabolism of the host cell, may promote its proliferation with an accompanying accumulation of genetic lesions, change the activity of proteins that have a suppressive effect on oncogenes, or integrate their genetic material into the genome of the host cell and with various mechanisms to bring about cell turnover and neoplasm development [39].

The mechanisms by which oncogenic viruses induce oncogenic transformation vary, but all have important common features. For example, a virus particle is capable of bringing about transformation. All or part of the viral genome remains in the transformed cells and this genome is expressed in these cells. Transformation is a result of the degeneration of normal cellular growth signals.

Studies of the oncogenic activity of proteins encoded by oncogenic viruses, especially DNA viruses, have greatly contributed to elucidating the role of retinoblastoma (Rb) proteins and the repressor gene p53 as regulators of cell growth. DNA oncoproteins of oncogenic viruses act to block the action of these two key proteins, thereby prompting a dormant cell to enter the S phase. Oncoproteins that target Rb and p53 are encoded by human tumor viruses, but they do so *via* distinct and distinct methods [40]. Telomerase reverse transcriptase [41–43], cytoplasmic PI3K–AKT–Mtor [44], nuclear factor-κB (NF-κB) [45], β-catenin (also called CTNNB1) [46] and interferon signaling pathways [47] are other common targets that play roles in carcinogenesis for tumor viruses (**Figure 5**).

The tumor suppressor gene TP53 is located on chromosome 17p13 and encodes the nuclear protein p53 (transcription factor), which is involved in maintaining the

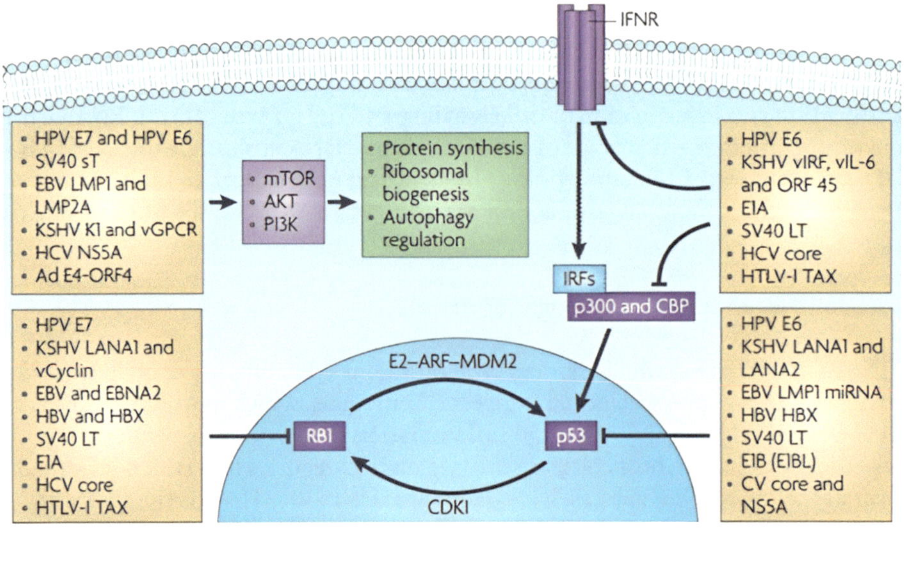

Figure 5.
Common cellular targets for unrelated tumor virus oncoproteins [7].

integrity of the genome and is responsible for the smooth functioning of repair mechanisms in case of DNA damage. It plays an important role in the regulation of the cell cycle and in the decisions that lead to apoptosis, cell differentiation and DNA damage repair [18, 48]. It causes cell cycle arrest in the G1 phase, allowing DNA repair or, in case of severe DNA damage, induces apoptosis-inducing factors. Thus, it is ensured that the mutated DNA is not duplicated and for this reason, the p53 gene is also called the "guardian of the genome". It promotes apoptosis by increasing Bax gene expression and decreasing bcl-2 gene. Mutated forms of p53 have altered functionality and may inactivate the natural (wild type) protein [17, 49]. Even in the absence of mutations, p53 can be inactivated through other mechanisms such as its binding to the E6 viral protein of oncogenic strains of HPV leading to its proteolysis [50].

Another tumor suppressor gene is INK4-ARF, whose protein product, protein p16, acts as an inhibitor of the cyclin-dependent kinases CDK4 and CDK6, preventing the cell from entering the S phase of the cell cycle and thereby controlling cell proliferation [26]. When the gene loses its function, together with overexpression of cyclin D1, the activity of CDK4 and CDK6 kinases is enhanced, resulting in increased cell proliferation. Inactivation of the gene can be through mutations, losses or methylation of the gene promoter [26, 51, 52]. Loss of p16 has been found in 63% of oral squamous cell carcinomas and in 59% of precancerous lesions of the same region, suggesting that this is an event that occurs early in carcinogenesis [53]. In HPV-positive oropharyngeal tumors, it has been found that the functional inactivation of the Rb pathway through the viral protein E7 induces the overexpression of p16 and therefore this protein has been proposed as a marker for neoplasms of the region [54]. Loss of p16 is also associated with poorer prognosis [26, 54].

Additionally, the ability to understand mutation in relation to viral infection provides an additional physiological dimension to the evolution of viral replication and the strategy by which one can examine mutation. Similarly, the reproduction and study of oncogenes in RNA oncogenic viruses were of great importance for the investigation of the course of transduction signals that connect the cell membrane with the regulation of the genetic apparatus in the cell nucleus. Perhaps the most important thing is that the oncogenes that were recruited by RNA oncogenic viruses encode proteins that are involved in almost all stages of the signal transduction pathway. Unlike the oncogenes of DNA oncogenes, those of RNA oncogenes are not necessarily viral genes, rather, they are cellular genes that the viruses acquired during their replication in cells, rendering them incapable of replication. The ability of cellular proteins to become trapped in the viral genome, change course and be transferred into a form that can alter the developmental properties of the cell is one of the most important events in the course of cell transformation. The power of this approach is fantastic, judging by the number of genes identified to date.

One external element that is very significant in predicting whether a cancer develops following exposure to a possible tumor virus is immunity [7]. This is seen in males with mutations in the signaling lymphocytic activation molecule-associated protein (SAP), which follows an EBV infection and results in immunodeficiency and X-linked lymphoproliferative disease. The significance of immunology in regulating the manifestation of a viral malignancy is further demonstrated by Kaposi's sarcoma, which was initially reported in 1872. Although KSHV and humans co-specited 80 million years ago, only about 3% of healthy North Americans are infected. Prior to the AIDS pandemic, KSHV produced fewer than three occurrences of Kaposi's sarcoma annually per million persons in the US. However, as immune suppression from the

HIV pandemic emerged, the incidence of Kaposi's sarcoma among AIDS patients increased tens of thousands of times.

Oncogenic viruses contribute to carcinogenesis by altering host epigenomes and using host epigenetic machinery. Chromatin alterations and processes that affect gene regulation without altering the DNA sequence itself are included in the field of epigenetics. In order to control viral gene expression, divide their genomes into daughter cells and preserve viral latency in order to elude the host's immune system, viruses make use of host epigenetic modifiers. The growing list of such mechanisms includes non-coding RNAs (ncRNAs), DNA methylation and histone post-translational modifications (PTMs). The impacts of virally mediated epigenetic changes on cancer pathology are: (1) epithelial-to-mesenchymal transition, (2) escape from apoptosis, (3) altered cellular metabolism, (4) angiogenesis, (5) inflammation and (6) generation of genomic instability [55]. **Table 2** highlights virally induced epigenetic modifications that are clearly associated with cancer pathogenesis.

3.3 RNA oncogenic viruses

RNA oncoviruses played an important role in establishing paradigms that extend beyond virology to form the foundation of modern cancer biology. At the beginning

Oncogenic virus	Oncoprotein	Mechanism	Impact on Host Epigenome	Impact on Cancer Pathology
EBV	• LMP1	• Direct interaction with *DNMT1* promoter, driving its overexpression	• Hypermethylation of numerous promoters, including *CDH1*	• Epithelial–Mesenchymal Transition (EMT), metabolic reprogramming
	• EBNA3A and EBNA3C	• Recruit PRC2 to *BIM* promoter	• Repression of *BIM* transcription *via* H3K27me3 and DNA methylation	• Escape from apoptosis
HPVs (high-risk)	• E6	• Downregulation of miR-34a	• Upregulation of LDHA	• Metabolic reprogramming
	• E7	• Neomorphic LDHA generation *via* Reactive Oxygen Species (ROS) production	• Production of α-HB increasing H3K79me3 and activating Wnt signaling	• Metabolic reprogramming, increased cell proliferation
		• Promotes *EZH2* expression in cervical cancer	• Increased deposition of repressive H3K27me3 mark	• Escape from apoptosis and increased cell proliferation
	• E6 and E7	Upregulation of *DNMT1* expression	• Hypermethylation of numerous promoters, including *CDH1*	• EMT
HBV	• HBx	• Upregulation of DNMT1 *via* p16 promoter hypermethylation	• Hypermethylation of numerous promoters, including *CDH1*	• EMT
		• HBx-LINE1 acts as sponge for miR-122	• Lack of miR-122 expression	• Inflammation
HCV	• HCV core protein	• Activates transcription of *DNMT1* and *DNMT3B*	• Hypermethylation of numerous promoters, including *CDH1*	• EMT

Oncogenic virus	Oncoprotein	Mechanism	Impact on Host Epigenome	Impact on Cancer Pathology
HTLV-1	• HBZ	• Sequesters FOX03a and binds to p300/CBP to promote their dissociation from the *BIM* promoter in ATL	• Repression of BIM *via* deposition of H3K27me3 by PRC2 (EZH2 is upregulated in ATL)	• Escape from apoptosis
		• Increases miR17 and miR21 expression, resulting in downregulation of OBFC2A	• Increased expression of oncogenic miRNAs	• Genomic instability
	• Tax	• Promotes EZH2 activity in ATL	• Increased deposition of repressive H3K27me3 mark	• Escape from apoptosis
KSHV	• LANA	• Binds to TβRII promoter, resulting in DNA methylation and H4 deacetylation	• Inhibition of TGF-β signaling	• Angiogenesis
	• vFLIP and vCyclin	• Upregulates miR-17-92, which targets *SMAD2*	• Inhibition of TGF-β signaling	• Angiogenesis
	• VIRF1	• Upregulates circARFGEF, which acts as a sponge for miR-125a-3p	• Increases expression of *GLRX3*	• Angiogenesis
MCPyV	Small T-antigen	• Binds to L-MYC to recruit EP400 chromatin remodeling complex	• Transcriptional regulation of multiple genes	• Cell viability and stemness

Table 2.
Viral oncoprotein-mediated epigenetic processes and their effects on the host epigenome [55].

of the last century, with the discovery of the Rous sarcoma virus, by Payton Rous, that the virus causes cancer and specifically sarcomas in poultry; RNA oncogenic viruses were placed in a group of microorganisms with special characteristics. These features were the transcription of RNA into DNA, the integration of DNA into the cellular genome (into the cell's chromosome) and the expression of this integrated DNA (provirus) under viral transcriptional control. Reverse transcription gave the group of viruses the name retroviruses. Further infection with these viruses is based on their integration into the cellular genome and lack of cytotoxic activity. The viral genome is passed down as a set of Mendelian markers after being established in the germline. Two aspects of the viral growth cycle that directly affect integration into the host genome are particularly significant for oncogenesis. The first is the integrated provirus's capacity to take up and transfer cellular genetic material, and the second is the insertion activation of cellular genes [56, 57]. Proviruses may integrate into the cellular genome at additional locations. The integrated transcript resembles a biological gene, with the exception that the viral Long Terminal Repeat (LTR) typically contains sequences that regulate transcription.

Retrovirus infection is permanent as the provirus never disappears from the chromosome. Retroviruses cause tumors and transform cells by three different mechanisms, while most of them achieve tumorigenesis through oncogene actions. Retroviruses form two different groups: those that carry an oncogene in their genome and are called transducers, and those that lack an oncogene but have the ability to transform in the vicinity of a cellular oncogene (these viruses are referred to as cis-activators). The oncogenes identified in retroviruses and which were the first group of genes involved in cancer development are damaged cellular genes called oncogenes (v-oncogenes), as opposed to normal genes called proto-oncogenes or cellular genes (c-oncogenes). For example, the ras and jun oncogenes are found in eukaryotic cells from yeast to humans. All oncogenes act through protein products called oncoproteins. That is, oncogenes instruct cells to make a protein that greatly stimulates cell growth and division. The increased rate of growth and proliferation also results in the creation of mutations involving DNA repair genes, oncogenes and various other tumor suppressor genes (tumor suppressor genes). The accumulation of mutations (damages) results in the formation of tumors.

In addition to cellular proto-oncogenes and viral oncogenes that are involved in the creation of cancer, there are also repressor genes, which are normal genes that instruct the cell to produce proteins that inhibit cell division. These genes are the "brakes" that stop uncontrolled proliferation at an uncontrolled rate. The loss of a tumor suppressor gene has deleterious consequences for the growth of the cell as it allows the cell to proliferate uncontrollably and continuously. It is now known that the loss of function of the p53 gene, as a result of a mutation or deletion, coincides with the development of cancer [58]. In fact, research indicates that the great majority of human malignancies may be caused by a lack of p53 gene function. Retroviruses have been found to include over 30 transduced oncogenes [59]. Recombination during the second round of replication results in the integration of the cellular gene into the viral genome, and the potential induction of a provirus upstream of a proto-oncogene may result in chimeric virus-cell transcripts. This capture frequently results in the loss of viral genes, resulting in viruses that are dysfunctional and reliant on a helper virus within the same cell to deliver the viral functions required for reproduction. Highly transforming retroviruses that carry oncogenes do not induce a significant number of tumors, and it is doubtful whether these viruses can survive for a long time in nature due to their defective phenotype. Retroviruses can thus be classified into the category of simple viruses or into the category of composites based on the organization of the genome. Only simple retroviruses seem to induce cellular genes while complex viruses such as HIV and HTLV do not have this ability. Perhaps the more complex and genetically organized a virus is, the more difficult it is for it to tolerate foreign inserts (DNA) and to be able to maintain its shape and reproduce. As previously stated, an oncogene is released from the impact of cellular restrictions and expressed in transduced cells under the viral LTR's control once it has been incorporated into the viral genome. Another possibility is that the transducing retrovirus infects a cell type that lacks the regulators necessary to govern the proto-oncogene since it does not express it. The target cell undergoes cellular transformation as a result of this confluence of circumstances, namely the overexpression or improper expression of a changed gene linked to development. Transgenic oncogene-carrying retroviruses alter cells *in vitro* and cause cancers in animals after a brief latent phase. Some viruses (mouse mammary tumor virus, avian leukosis virus, etc.) do not carry an oncogene and yet can create tumors in animals, and they achieve this by inserting a provirus near a cellular proto-oncogene a process called proviral insertional mutagenesis. Gene expression is altered when a provirus inserts strong promoter and enhancer sequences into the nearby gene site [60]. Oncogene-free retroviruses can replicate, do not change cells *in vitro*, and develop tumors after a protracted dormant period *in vivo*. There is replication of these viruses during latency before the tumor even develops and possibly a fortuitous event placing the provirus in close proximity to the cellular oncogene. This fact apparently gives the cell an advantage in its growth and ensures its survival while over time, more genetic changes accumulate. Tumors arising from a long latent period are cloned, indicating the existence of events that cooperate to create a transformed cell capable of uncontrolled proliferation and tumorigenesis.

It is now well established that a virus's capacity to multiply and infect a significant number of cells within a target organ raises the possibility that a cell's growth-related gene will be subverted. However, studies with oncogenic viruses have shown that the same oncogene is not activated by the introduction of the provirus in all samples of a given tumor type, which reveals that different biochemical changes at the cellular level can lead to the same pathoanatomical alteration [60]. However, there are some examples where a given oncogene is frequently altered such as c-myc in avian leukemia and N-myc in woodchuck hepatitis [61].

3.4 DNA oncogenic viruses

DNA oncogenes are a family of viruses (**Table 3**) with a very diverse structure, genomic organization and replication strategy. DNA oncogenic viruses, in contrast to RNA oncogenic viruses, lack a reverse transcriptase (reverse transcriptase) because they probably do not need it since with their DNA they can be directly involved in cellular DNA. It has been observed that some DNA viruses are responsible for tumor

Virus family	Envelope present	Capsid symmetry	Virion size (nm)	DNA MW ($\times 10^6$)	DNA structure[1]	Medically important viruses
Parvovirus	No	Icosahedral	22	2	SS, linear	B19 virus
Polyomavirus	No	Icosahedral	45	3	DS, circular, supercoiled	JC virus, BK virus
Papillomavirus	No	Icosahedral	55	5	DS, circular, supercoiled	Human papillomavirus
Adenovirus	No	Icosahedral	75	23	DS, linear	Adenovirus
Hepadnavirus	Yes	Icosahedral	42	1.5	DS, incomplete circular	Hepatitis B virus
Herpesvirus	Yes	Icosahedral	100[2]	100-150	DS, linear	Herpes simplex virus, varicella-zoster virus, cytomegalovirus, Epstein-Barr virus
Poxvirus	Yes	Complex	250 × 400	125–185	DS, linear	Smallpox virus, molluscum contagiosum virus

[1]SS = single-stranded; DS = double-stranded.
[2]The herpesvirus nucleocapsid is 100 nm, but the envelope varies in size. The entire virus can be as large as 200 nm in diameter.

Table 3.
Classification of DNA Viruses [62].

induction in their natural host including humans, while in other cases, they induce transformation in cells *in vitro* and create tumors in laboratory animals.

These properties are opposite to those retroviruses where cellular oncogenes are transferred by them and thus DNA oncogene viruses are able to carry out a productive infection, that is, infection of a cell that will lead to the production of new virus particles directly and without the intervention of another helper virus.

Transformation of a cell will occur under non-permissive conditions in which the viral replication pathway is inefficient. Oncoviruses' capacity to induce a quiescent (non-proliferating) cell to enter the cell cycle is reflected in oncogenic events mediated by their DNA oncoproteins. For instance, a well-differentiated epithelial cell lining the upper respiratory system is a normal cell that an adenovirus targets. Both viral and cellular DNA are scarce in this cell since it has not begun the cell cycle. Particularly during the cell cycle, deoxyribonucleotide levels are strictly controlled and rise during the S phase [63]. Effective viral replication depends on the virus's capacity to cause the cell to enter S phase, which creates an environment conducive to DNA replication. Induction of S phase by the virus depends on viral genes that otherwise lead to transformation.

Thus, if the infection does not proceed to completion, either due to non-acceptance by the cell, or as a result of viral transformation, which arrests the growth of the virus, the breakdown of the control of cell growth that was intended to prepare the cell for viral infection perhaps leading to the development of a transformed cell.

Early and mature phases of a viral infection are distinguished by the interval between viral gene expression and DNA replication. The structural elements of the virion are found in the products of mature genes, whereas the early genes often produce proteins that prime the infected cell for viral DNA replication. The oncogenic transformation is caused by the early gene products of DNA oncogenic viruses. Small DNA oncogenes rely on the host cell's machinery to replicate their viral DNA due to their minimal genetic content. Nonstructural proteins encoded by viruses cause dormant cells to enter S phase, which provides enzymes and a conducive environment for DNA replication.

The binding of oncoproteins to the repressor proteins, as already mentioned, namely p53 and pRb, is an important factor in the effect of small DNA oncogenes on host cells [64, 65]. The significance of pRb and p53 in cell growth and the need for viruses to evade this regulation are demonstrated by the fact that different DNA oncogene viruses express distinct oncoproteins that target these two proteins. In cells infected with this virus, the p53 protein was found to be a cellular protein attached to the SV40 T-antigen. A few years later it was discovered that normal p53 was not oncogenic but was in fact a suppressive protein which arrested cell growth [66, 67]. A second repressor protein, the product of the retinoblastoma gene, pRb, was identified as one of several cellular proteins associated with the adenovirus early region 1A (E1A) oncoprotein in cells transformed with an adenovirus [67]. The oncogenic viruses that have been studied in recent years, the oncoproteins of the oncogenic viruses and their interactions with cellular proteins, are shown in **Table 4**.

The following is the simplified scenario for this interaction: The transcription factor E2F is often bound by pRb during the G1 phase of the cell cycle. Cyclin-dependent kinases phosphorylate pRb, releasing E2F, which activates the production of growth-stimulating genes necessary for the cell to start DNA synthesis. T-antigens release active E2F by causing the pRb-E2F complex to disintegrate spontaneously. By stopping the advancement of the cell cycle or triggering apoptosis in response to abnormal proliferative signals, DNA damage, or cellular stress, p53 protects the integrity of the

Virus	Viral oncoprotein	Cellular targets
SV40	Large T-antigen	P53, pRb
	Small antigen	PP2A
HPV	E6	P53 *via* E6AP, DLG, MAGI-1, MUPP1
	E7	pRb
Adeno	E1A	pRb
	E1B-55 K	P53
Adeno9	E4ORF1	DLG, MAGI-1, MUPP1
BPV	E5	PDGFβ receptor
HBV	HBx	P53, DDB1
Polyma	Large T-antigen	pRb
	Middle T-antigen	c-Src, PI3-k, PLC-γ, She
	Small T-antigen	PP2A

Table 4.
DNA virus oncoproteins and cellular protein interactions [68].

cellular genome. It plays a crucial role in controlling a complicated cycle that involves other proteins in the cell [69]. Because T-antigens deactivate p53, cells that have been improperly activated by the release of E2F are able to evade p53 regulation, enter S phase, survive and reproduce viral DNA.

DNA oncogenic viruses show different ways to achieve the same result, that is, sudden biological change of p53. Viral oncoproteins bind p53 through different sequences. When the T-antigens of the oncogenic virus SV40, for example, bind to p53, they block its binding capacity, while E6 of HPV degrades it and E1B-55 K of adenoviruses interferes with the function of trans, that is, through other genes in other places of the cell. By combining with viral oncoproteins, these same oncogenic viruses render pRb inactive. For instance, a sequence of amino acids seen in the T-antigen of SV40, E7 of HPV and E1A of adenovirus is crucial for binding to pRb. When it comes to the hypophosphorylated form of pRb—the type that binds E2F and is distinguished from the hyperphosphorylated version—viral proteins show exceptional selectivity. The only viral oncoprotein that can interact with both pRb and p53 is SV40 T-antigen. It should be mentioned that DNA oncogenic viruses and their proteins may also target other different cellular proteins, as this was recently demonstrated with the E6 protein of HPV viruses belonging to high-risk HPV types.

In the last 30 years, with the studies done with oncogenic viruses everything has changed about the genesis of cancer. Scientists working on chemical carcinogenesis, oncogenic viruses or other carcinogens followed a parallel path, each group believing that their own system was the most unique and correct. But everything changed when it was discovered that the genes from lung and bladder cancer were homologous to the ras genes that had already been identified and identified as oncogenes in viruses that caused sarcoma in mice. In parallel investigations with carcinogens that created tumors in the persistent, it was observed that these carcinogens activated the H-ras gene [70]. It was now clear that somatic mutations, chemical carcinogens or viruses all changed the same cellular proto-oncogenes. Several oncogenes that had previously been identified and detected in RNA oncogenic viruses were discovered to be mutated in human cancers in a short amount of time. One such example is the myc gene in leukemias [71]. The integration of human and viral oncology was finalized with the following identification of suppressor genes. Human cancer research currently focuses a lot of attention on oncogenes and suppressor genes, and complements to these two gene groups—which are linked to cancer and have no counterparts in oncogenic viruses—have been found. Through the use of viruses, it was proven that changed cellular regulatory genes are the biological basis of cancer.

Oncogenic virus	Genome	Family	Associated cancer types	Global infection prevalence	Global attributable fraction
EBV	dsDNA ~170 kb	Her-pesviridae	• BL	• >90%	• BL (~55%)
			• HL		• HL (~46–58%)
			• ENKTL		• ENKTL (100%)
			• DLBCL		• DLBCL (~4–13%)
			• NPC		• NPC (~85%)
			• GC		• GC (~8–10%)
			• Pediatric		• Pediatric LMS (LD)
			• LMS		• All cancers (~1.5%)
HPVs	dsDNA ~8 kb	Papillo-maviridae	• CC	• ~75%	• CC (>95%)
			• HNSCC		• HNSCC (~30% oropharyngeal, ~2% oral, ~2% laryngeal)
			• AC		• AC (anal ~88%, vulvar ~25%, vaginal ~78%, penile ~50%)
			• EV-associated		• EV-associated (LD)
					• All cancers (~4.5%)
HBV	dsDNA ~3.2 kb	Hepadna-viridae	• HCC	• ~4%	• HCC (~56%)
HCV	ssRNA ~9.6 kb	Flaviviridae	• HCC	• ~1%	• HCC (~20%)
			• NHL		• NHL (~3%)
HTLV-1	ssRNA ~9 kb	Retroviridae	• ATL	• <1%	• ATL (100%)
KSHV	dsDNA ~165 kb	Herpesviridae	• KS	• <10%	• KS (100%) •
			• NHL		• NHL (LD)
MCPyV	dsDNA ~5.4 kb	Polyomaviridae	• MCC	• ~80%	• MCC (~36–80%)

Human papillomavirus (HPV), Epstein-Barr virus (EBV), hepatitis B virus (HBV), hepatitis C virus (HCV), human T-cell leukemia virus type 1 (HTLV-1), Kaposi's sarcoma-associated herpesvirus (KSHV), Merkel cell polyomavirus (MCPyV), double-stranded (ds), single-stranded (ss) and kb Burkitt's lymphoma (BL), Hodgkin's lymphoma (HL), extranodal natural killer/T-cell lymphoma (ENKTL), nasopharyngeal carcinoma (NPC), gastric carcinoma (GC), leiomyosarcoma (LMS), cervical cancer (CC), head and neck squamous cell carcinoma (HNSCC), anogenital carcinoma (AC), epidermodysplasia verruciformis (EV), hepatocellular carcinoma (HCC), adult T-cell leukemia/lymphoma (ATL), Kaposi's sarcoma (KS), non-Hodgkin's lymphoma (NHL), Merkel cell carcinoma (MCC) and lacking data (LD).

Table 5.
Oncogenic viruses and their associated malignancies [55].

There are currently six viruses that are blamed for human cancer, and they are hepatitis B virus (HBV), hepatitis C virus (HCV), some strains of human papillomavirus (HPV), Epstein-Barr virus (HBV), AIDS virus (HIV) and human immunodeficiency virus type 1 (HTLV-1). In addition, Kaposi's sarcoma-associated virus (HHV8) is classified as a probable human carcinogen.

A large number of viruses isolated from monkeys and other animals cause cancer, and these animals have been used as models to study the mechanisms of viral carcinogenesis that form the basis of what we know today. It is believed that 15% of human cancers have a viral etiology [72]. The rate of virus-related cancer is three times higher in developing countries and this reflects the high prevalence of viral infection. Some viruses such as HBV are associated with one type of cancer, while others such as EBV are associated with several types (**Table 5**). These differences likely reflect the tissue (cell) tropism of a particular virus.

4. Oncogenic viruses in head and neck cancers

4.1 Human papillomavirus (HPV) and head and neck cancer

4.1.1 Introduction

Human papilloma viruses (HPV) are small DNA viruses that grow and multiply inside epithelial cells (**Figure 6**). They present a specific tropism for the covering epithelium of the skin and mucous membrane, in which they cause hyperplastic and tumorous changes [73]. HPV belongs to the *Papillomavirus* genus, Papovaviridae family. Based on their capacity to cause cancer, more than 200 HPV genotypes have been divided into low-risk and high-risk categories. Twelve HPV types—16, 18, 31, 33, 35, 39, 45, 51, 52, 56, 58 and 59—are categorized as carcinogenic to humans by the International Agency for Research on Cancer (IARC) [74]. The lengthy control section in HPV's genome, which contributes significantly to genomic variation, makes it easier for the virus to spread through direct sexual contact. The E1, E2, E4, E5, E6, E7 and E8 genes responsible for cell transformation and replication, as well as late genes for viral particle assembly, make up the viral genome [75].

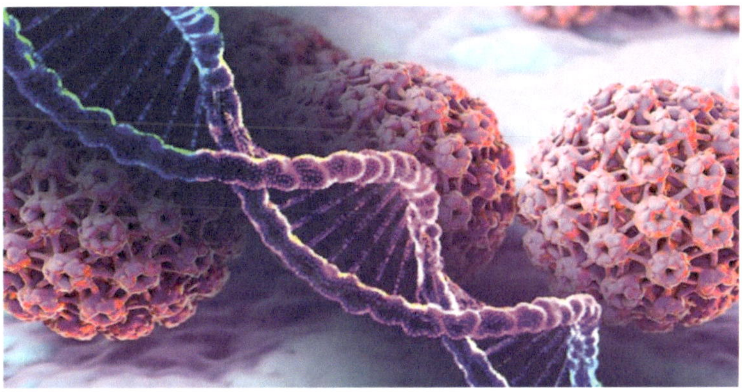

Figure 6.
Human papillomavirus. Credit: University of Maryland School of Medicine.

There is a considerable range in the prevalence of HPV-associated HNC, from 20 to 80%. Geographical disparities, a range of demographic characteristics and variations in the sensitivity and specificity of HPV detection techniques are some of the causes of this large variation [11]. These variations show how difficult it is to comprehend how HPV affects HNC in various groups and how consistent diagnostic standards are required to properly evaluate and treat this worldwide health issue. Worldwide, HPV is a sexually transmitted infection that affects both men and women and has been extensively researched in the literature. Associations between HPV infection and various cancers have been established, ranging from penile, cervical, vaginal and vulvar cancers to HNC, particularly oropharyngeal cancer [76].

HPV predominantly targets basal cells to start infection, and it infects epithelial cells through minor abrasions and wounds. The virus can linger in the cellular environment for extended periods of time due to this ineffective infection [77]. Acquisition, persistence, precancerous development and invasion stages make up the viral life cycle, and a chronic infection raises the risk of cancer by a large margin. Because HPV compartmentalizes gene expression at different cellular levels and preserves its genome in the form of episomes, it is crucial to comprehend its long-term infectious potential rather than its pathogenicity [78]. The virus uses host cell

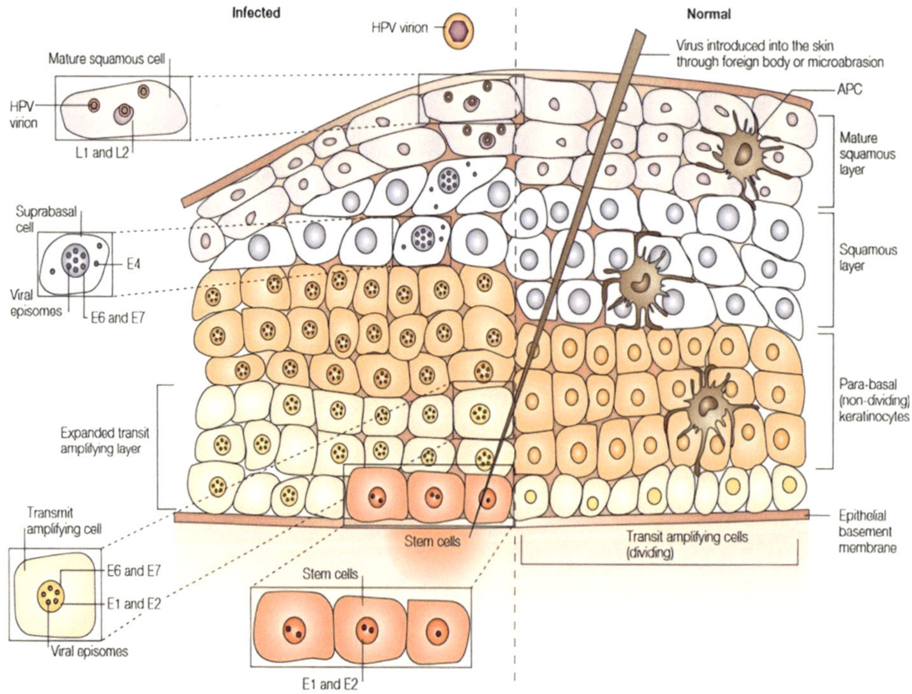

Figure 7.

The primary stages of the papillomavirus life cycle are located in the squamous epithelium. Architecture of cervical stratified squamous epithelial cells and post-infection expression of human papillomavirus (HPV) proteins. After dividing along the basement membrane, daughter cells of epithelial stem cells mature vertically through the epithelium without undergoing additional division (right side). Viral nonstructural protein expression happens once HPV is introduced into stem cells in the epithelium's basal layer. These proteins control the vertical expansion of the dividing-cell population and the delayed and incomplete differentiation of epithelial cells. Only the outermost layers of the epithelium produce mature virions, and viral proteins are expressed in a sequential manner with differentiation as demonstrated. Intraepithelial antigen-presenting cells (APCs) are depleted in the HPV-infected epithelium [79].

replication processes and only weakly expresses the E1 and E2 genes after entering basal epithelial cells (**Figure 7**). In suprabasal cells, HPV expresses the E1 and E2 genes along with the E6 and E7 genes, altering cell cycle regulators and resulting in cell immortalization during the non-spreading phase while avoiding immune detection [80]. Amplification of the viral genome and creation of new virions are encouraged by early gene expression, particularly that of E4 and E5 [6].

In many cases, sexually acquired HPV infection is eliminated by the immune system. However, once HPVs are integrated into the host genome, an important phase of HPV-induced oncogenesis begins. Unique oncogenes expressed by integrated HPV impact cell cycle control mechanisms, cause genomic instability, and ultimately contribute to the progression of cancer [81]: HPV E6 inhibits apoptosis by disrupting p53 *via* E6AP, while E7 targets pRb for abnormal cell growth and degradation, promoting apoptosis (**Figure 8**). Additionally, E6 interacts with c-myc to increase h-TERT levels, which further contributes to cell transformation and an endless lifespan [6].

4.1.2 HPV's role in oropharyngeal cancer

The significant increase in HPV (+) OPSCC over the last 15 years in non-smoking and young patients [83] reflects the increasing prevalence of HPV infection in the oral cavity as a causative factor, possibly due to changes in sexual behavior [84].

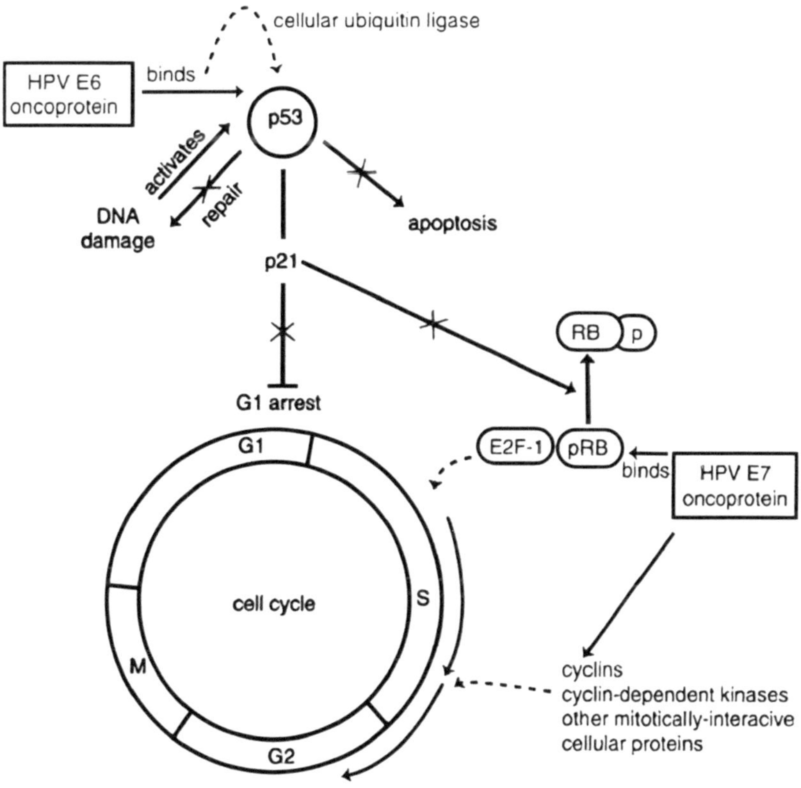

Figure 8.
Oncogenic HPV pathogenesis. The multifunctional proteins encoded by the HPV E6 and E7 genes bind mainly to the cellular p53 and pRB proteins, interfere with their functions and change cell cycle regulatory pathways, ultimately causing cellular transformation [82].

According to the literature, the detected number of HPV (+) oropharyngeal neoplasms is constantly increasing, constituting >50% of the total number of head and neck neoplasms [85] and 25.6% of oropharyngeal squamous cell carcinomas worldwide are associated with HPV infection; however, variation in virus positivity rates is observed depending on the geographic region [84]. Specifically, in North America HPV(+) squamous cell carcinomas of the oropharynx range from 56% in Japan, 52% in Australia, 45% in Southern and Western Europe, 39% in Eastern Europe, 38% in Northern Europe at 17% and in the rest of the world at 13% [84].

The observed decline in tobacco use in the US, which is an established risk factor for the development of HPV, led to a parallel decrease in the incidence of HPV(−) cancers by 50% [86]. In contrast, the incidence of HPV (+) squamous cell carcinomas of the oropharynx increased by 225% in the period 1988–2004 [65] with a similar trend recorded in both Europe and Australia [87].

The incidence of HPV (+) squamous cell carcinomas of the oropharynx is higher among middle-aged men (40–59 years), non-smokers with higher socioeconomic status and multiple partners, with a higher rate of metastatic lymph node disease at diagnosis. In particular, patients with HPV(+) squamous cell carcinomas of the oropharynx are less likely to be associated with smoking and alcohol abuse, while having an average of more than 8 to 10 sexual partners compared to those diagnosed with HPV(−) neoplasms [88]. The possibility of HPV involvement is two to three times greater in precancerous lesions of the oral cavity and four to five times greater in invasive oral cancer than in normal mucosa [53].

Tissue-specific factors like epithelial structure, microflora composition, immune response and environmental influences contribute to differences in how HPV-associated cancers develop and progress in these different anatomical sites, despite the fact that the basic mechanisms of HPV infection and viral life cycle are similar in cervical and oral epithelial cells. It is yet unknown what specific factors contribute to the persistence of oral HPV infection. In the cell, HPV typically begins as a circular episomal form before changing to a linear form and integrating into the host DNA. Embedded HPVs are usually located in cervical cancer [89]; HPV integration in HNC does not occur at a single site but at multiple splice breakpoints [90]; studies on HNC cell lines suggest that these breakpoints are associated with genomic instability, an important feature of virus-induced carcinogenesis. Integration further promotes cell transformation by increasing HPV E6 and E7 expression [91].

Infection of the oral epithelium with HPV is possible through oropharyngeal contact and is associated with high-risk sexual practices, which facilitate repeated exposure to the virus. The majority of HCVs caused by HPV infection originate from the oropharyngeal mucosa and mainly from the parsopharyngeal tonsils and the base of the tongue (mainly from the lingual tonsil). Specifically, most HPV (+) tonsillar neoplasms are located in the tonsillar crypts, which appear to be vulnerable to HPV infection [75]. In contrast, HPV (−) neoplasms or neoplasms due to smoking arise in the surface epithelium. Crypts are dips of the squamous epithelium in the lymphatic tissue of the tonsil and can harbor non-pathogenic as well as pathogenic microorganisms. The reticular squamous epithelium covering the tonsillar crypts is structured in such a way as to allow direct contact with the lymphoid tissue and the transfer of exogenous antigens from the external environment of the oropharynx to the lymphoid tissue of the tonsils.

In addition, the basement membrane is partially permeable allowing the passage of lymphocytes and antigen-presenting cells into the basal layer of the epithelium [92]. In the transition zone of the cervix, HPV infection requires disruption of the squamous epithelium continuity, for viral particles to enter the exposed basement membrane. In contrast, the reticular configuration of the epithelium of the tonsillar crypts contributes to the exposure of the basement membrane to viral pathogens, without the need for mucosal microtrauma [92].

The microanatomy of the epithelium of tonsillar crypts is likely to contribute to some clinical features of HPV (+) tonsillar carcinomas, as well as the tendency of even small carcinomas to present as locally advanced metastases.

Although HPV (+) AKKT patients are diagnosed with advanced disease, they show higher rates of treatment response, overall survival and disease progression-free survival than HPV (−) patients [75]. In several clinical trials with advanced oropharyngeal neoplasms, the improvement in survival is two to three times greater in HPV(+) than in HPV(−) neoplasms, with approximately 75% of this improvement attributable to the biological behavior of HPV(+) cancers and 25% in healthy patients. Accordingly, HPV positivity has been recognized as the strongest independent prognostic factor for oropharyngeal squamous cell carcinomas.

4.1.3 Implication of HPV infection in laryngeal cancer

HPV is recognized to play a part in genital and oropharyngeal cancers, but its function in laryngeal cancer is less evident. While alcohol use and smoking continue to be the primary risk factors for laryngeal cancer, HPV is more common in younger individuals and non-smokers. Of the several HPV subtypes, HPV-16 and HPV-18 are commonly found in laryngeal cancer, and HPV-16 is highly correlated with the occurrence and outcome of cancer [93]. A systematic review and meta-analysis was carried out 10 years ago by Li et al. [94] to look at the connection between HPV infection and laryngeal cancer. The overall HPV prevalence in laryngeal cancer tissue was found to be 28.0%, and high-risk HPV types were detected in 26.6%, especially HPV-16 in 19.8%. Gama et al. conducted a review and meta-analysis of 179 studies on HPV prevalence in LSCC covering 7347 cases was performed. The results revealed that HPV was found in 25% of cases and that the significant variation was mainly related to geographical factors rather than specific methods for HPV detection [95]. This underlines the important influence of geographical origin on the impact of HPV on the epidemiology of laryngeal cancer.

In normal laryngeal mucosa the virus isolation frequency is about 20% [96]. Of the benign papillomatous lesions of the larynx, HPV is isolated in around 10%. The virus serotypes responsible are 6 and 11. Although these are benign processes, newer studies report a 2% risk of malignant transformation [97]. The transformation takes place over a long period of time, 15–20 years, and it is considered that other factors such as smoking or alcohol consumption have a synergistic effect. Erkul et al. investigated the presence and potential prognostic role of HPV in LSCC [98]. Consequently, 26.02% of cases had HPV DNA found, and patients with HPV had a somewhat greater 3-year survival rate than those without HPV; however, these differences were not statistically significant. In contrast to earlier data, the study also highlighted a higher prevalence of high-risk HPV-16 in these malignancies [26]. The authors concluded that HPV might not be a reliable enough biomarker for diagnostic and prognostic purposes in LSCC in spite of these findings.

4.1.4 Mechanisms of improved response of HPV (+) HNSCCs to treatment

The improved response of HPV (+) HNSCCs to treatment is mainly attributed to the following mechanisms:

1. *Special characteristics* of the most commonly affected patient population, which are associated with fewer comorbidities, younger age and reduced tobacco exposure. The above factors contribute only 9% to the observed differences in overall survival and progression-free survival between HPV (+) and HPV (−) tumors.

2. *HPV-induced tumorigenesis* in the head and neck region involves a significantly smaller number of genetic changes compared to that not associated with the HPV virus. In particular, HPV (+) HNSCCs are less likely to have the mutant type of p53, high expression of epidermal growth factor receptor (EGFR) and chromosomal alterations of regions 3p, 9p and 17p [75, 99]. Recent molecular studies confirmed the different genetic profile of HPV (+) HNSCC and found more mutations in HPV (−) HNSCC than HPV-positive neoplasms, regardless of smoking history. These findings indicate that HPV-induced tumorigenesis is associated with a lesser degree of cell dysregulation, which contributes to a better response to treatment given the easier pathway to restore cell cycle normalization mechanisms.

3. *Response to treatment options*: HPV (+) oropharyngeal tumors respond better to induction platinum-based chemotherapy than HPV (−) tumors. It has also been observed that HPV (+) oropharyngeal cancers show an improved response to radiotherapy regardless of radiotherapy regimen, radiosensitizer or addition of chemotherapy. Data from the SEER (Surveillance, Epidemiology and End Results) database showed that the difference in survival between HPV (+) and HPV (−) squamous cell carcinoma of the oropharynx was higher for patients treated with radiation therapy [74]. HPV-positive cancer cell lines have been shown to exhibit increased apoptosis and reduced survival after irradiation or reduced DNA repair capacity.

4. *Immune surveillance*: The immune system plays an important role in viral carcinogenesis and an increased rate of virus-related malignancies is observed in immunocompromised patients. Therefore, the involvement of immunosurveillance in the clearance of HPV-induced disease is to be expected.

4.2 Epstein-Barr virus (EBV) and head and neck cancers

4.2.1 Introduction

EBV is a DNA human γ-herpesvirus that belongs to the genus Lymphocryptoviruses and is transmitted between individuals through close contact, specifically through the exchange of saliva, which is why EBV-related diseases were previously called “kissing diseases” (kissing disease) (**Figure 9**). Catalyst for the discovery of the virus was the contribution of the surgeon Denis Burkitt, who observed for the first time in the East African region, in the 1950s, a new form of childhood cancer, which today we know as Burkitt’s lymphoma (Burkitt’s lymphoma, BL). The remarkably high incidence of this type of cancer in Equatorial Africa, and the apparent influence of climatic factors in determining these areas, led Burkitt to hypothesize that some infectious agent was involved in the etiology of the cancer [100]. This discovery came to the attention of Tony Epstein, who, together with PhD candidate Yvonne Barr, succeeded in cultivating cell lines from cells derived from the blood of BL patients. Observation of these cell lines by electron microscopic methods

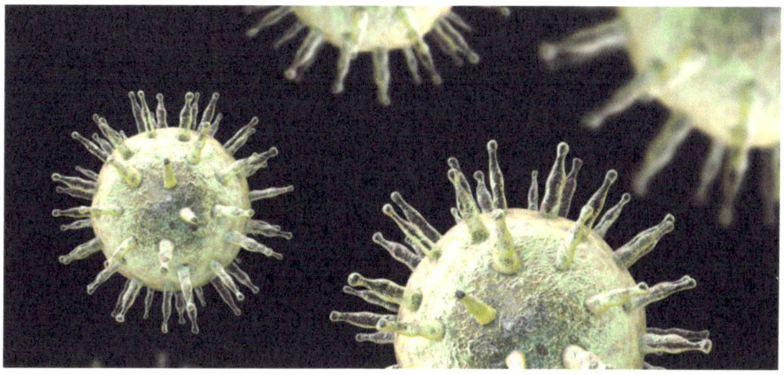

Figure 9.
Epstein-Barr virus.

revealed the existence of herpesvirus-like particles in a small percentage of the cells [101]. This agent was subsequently shown to be biologically and antigenically distinct from other members of the human herpesvirus family, and thus EBV was identified as the first potentially oncogenic human virus. The ability of EBV to immortalize peripheral blood B lymphocytes *in vitro*, and lead to their transformation into B lymphoblastoid cell lines (LCLs) [102], as well as studies in primates of Neo and of the Old World [103], established the association of EBV with malignant conditions. EBV is now the prototype of the γ-herpesvirus subfamily, which includes the genera γ1 or Lymphocryptoviruses (LCV) and γ2 or radinoviruses (RDV).

EBV is the only human LCV and KSHV (Kaposi's sarcoma-associated-19-herpesvirus) the only human RDV [104]. Given the similarity of the genomes of LCVs and RDVs and the restriction of occurrence of LCVs to primates, it appears that they evolved from some early RDV. The initial classification of the γ-herpesvirus subfamily was based on the biological properties of the viruses rather than similarities in genome organization. Thus, after adjustments to the systematic classification, EBV has been renamed as human herpes virus 4 (HHV4), although the term EBV still prevails in the literature.

4.2.2 Epidemiological evidence for EBV

Contrary to the initial association of EBV with a disease, which shows a specific geographic localization, seroepidemiological studies have shown that the virus is widespread, with over 95% of the human population worldwide appearing seropositive for it. In addition, virus can be isolated *in vitro* from lymphocyte cultures [105] or from pharyngeal washings of immunopositive individuals [106], indicating that EBV persists in individuals immunized against the virus.

In the United States and United Kingdom, 50% of children are infected before the age of 5. Seroepidemiological studies on the presence of IgG antibodies against the viral capsid antigen (VCA) complex show that the majority of children in the developing world are infected within the first 3 years of life, with this percentage reaching 100% of people, within the first decade. In these cases, infection is almost always asymptomatic and probably reflects transmission from the parent *via* the oral route.

In contrast, changing lifestyles in the developed Western world mean that nearly half of children remain HIV-negative even after their first decade of life and subsequently become infected with the virus through saliva exchange during adolescence or early childhood, phases of adulthood. Infection of an individual with EBV in this age range is responsible for the onset of infectious mononucleosis (IM) [107], a disease characterized by severe viral symptoms of long duration. About half of these infections are symptomatic, although usually only severe cases are finally diagnosed.

According to epidemiological studies, 5% of the human population in developed Western societies remains negative for EBV infection and constitutes a group of people from which rare cases of classical IM [108] or cases of iatrogenic mononucleosis arise, following transfusions or transplants [109].

Despite such a high percentage of EBV carriers, the infection remains asymptomatic in most cases. However, many times, EBV infection can lead to malignant conditions.

Thus, in our time, EBV is associated with 1% of all cancer cases worldwide, ranking fourth as an infectious agent in the frequency of related cancer cases. Its genome is detected in 30–90% of nasopharyngeal carcinomas. In stage I patients, the antibody titer is around 45%, while in stage IV, the percentage is 100%.

4.2.3 EBV's association with nasopharyngeal and other HNCs

EBV is arguably the most carcinogenic herpes virus. It contaminates about 90–95% of the adult human population worldwide and causes lifelong latent infection, mostly through saliva [110]. This extensive allocation suggests that it plays an important role in several cancers, including nasopharyngeal cancer, Burkitt's lymphoma, Hodgkin's lymphoma and gastric cancer. EBV is classified as a Group I carcinogen by IARC [12, 111].

EBV adopts a 'hit and run' tactic, manipulating host epigenetic procedures to start an oncogenic pathway even after the virus has been eliminated. Regardless of the virus's presence, this reprogramming causes genetic alterations in gene expression that impact the course of cancer [112]. Latent viral proteins, including EBV nuclear antigen (EBNA) and latent membrane proteins (LMPs), which disrupt cell function, promote proliferation and halt apoptosis, are responsible for the carcinogenic consequences of EBV [113]. About 80 genes and surface glycoproteins, including terminal repeats crucial for episome formation, are encoded by its linear double-stranded DNA genome [114]. The virus can affect B cells and epithelial cells by going into either a lysogenic or latent phase. By modifying cellular pathways *via* genes including EBNA1 and LMP1, EBV modifies cells during the latent period [115].

In HNCs, especially in nasopharyngeal and oral squamous cell carcinoma (OSCC), latent EBV proteins such as LMP1 stimulate uncontrolled growth by mimicking CD40 and tumor necrosis factor receptors [116]. While the role of EBV in B-cell malignancies is better understood, the mechanisms of EBV in epithelioid cell carcinomas are not yet clear, with ongoing studies showing that latency also exists in healthy epithelial cells [117]. The most popular theory for the role of Epstein-Barr virus in the malignant transformation of epithelial cells is that it affects the genetic material of the B lymphocytes, it enters and alters the protective mechanism of apoptosis or programmed cell death [118]. This effect of the virus on the mechanism of apoptosis is carried out mainly by changing the activity of the oncogene p-53 and bcl-2 [119, 120].

There are also studies that report detection of the virus in hypopharyngeal and esophageal cancers at rates of 5–85% depending of course on the geographical area. EBV is a possible risk factor because it has also been found in laryngeal cancer cells. EBV appears to encourage tumor growth despite its low frequency and challenging diagnosis in laryngeal carcinoma. The EBV genome and latent protein EBNA were originally discovered in malignant laryngeal cancer cells by Brichácek et al. [121]. EBV may be a risk factor or cofactor in the onset and spread of laryngeal cancer, according to a comprehensive review and meta-analysis by De Lima et al. [122]. However, because of the virus's low prevalence in LSCC and its difficulties in detection, its exact significance in this cancer type is still up for debate. The future burden of EBV-related cancer may be lessened with continued study into EBV-host interactions and the creation of tailored treatments.

4.3 Human herpesvirus 8's contribution in HNC

First discovered in 1994, human herpesvirus 8 (HHV-8)—also referred to as Kaposi's sarcoma-associated herpesvirus, or KSHV—is a significant oncogenic pathogen linked to HNC. Due to their compromised immune systems, HIV-positive people are more likely to develop Kaposi's sarcoma (KS), a malignant tumor that affects the mucosal tissue of the mouth and throat [123]. In contrast to other human herpes viruses, HHV-8 exhibits a unique geographic distribution, with low prevalence in other regions and the highest seroprevalence in Africa and the Mediterranean region [124].

HHV-8 exerts its oncogenic effects through viral proteins that establish latent infection in endothelial cells, disrupt cellular control mechanisms and promote uncontrolled cell proliferation and survival. Sundry transforming proteins are encoded from HHV-8, including latency-associated nuclear antigen (LANA), viral interleukin-6 and viral G protein-coupled receptor [125]. These proteins cause cell proliferation, angiogenesis and apoptosis suppression by activating signaling pathways such NF-κB, MAPK and PI3K/Akt. By evading immune detection and creating an environment that is conducive to tumor growth, the virus's ability to suppress the host immune response further raises the risk of carcinogenesis [126]. In addition to KS, HHV-8 is linked to multicentric Castleman disease (MCD) and primary effusion lymphoma (PEL), both of which can affect the head and neck region. PEL is a rare, aggressive B-cell lymphoma that mostly affects bodily cavities, while it can also appear in the mouth [127]. HHV-8 is found in lymphoid tissue in MCD, a lymphoproliferative disease that causes head and neck lymphadenopathy and accelerates the course of the illness [128]. Five LSCC patients had HHV-8, according to Güvenç et al.'s investigation of HHV-8 in relation to HPV in 47 of these patients. Both HHV-8 and HPV DNA were found in one instance, indicating that HHV-8 may also play a role in laryngeal carcinogenesis alongside HPV [129].

4.4 Relationship between others oncogenic herpesviruses and HNCs

The human herpesvirus 1 (HHV-1), also known as the herpes simplex virus 1 (HSV-1), primarily causes oral herpes by infecting nerve cells latently, though it can occasionally reactivate and result in recurring oral sores. Chronic inflammation and genetic changes in host cells are believed to be caused by HSV-1. It is thought to play a role in oral cancer development through induction. Regardless of the detection of viral markers in oral cancer tissue, studies on the relationship between HSV-1 and HNC have yielded contradictory results [130, 131]. Von Stebut et al., in a recent study, attempted to evaluate the association between HSV infection and HNC using TriNetX data. Their retrospective analysis included 249,272 patients and compared HSV infection status. The study found a considerable connection between HSV infection and lip cancer, with a striking hazard ratio of 1.17 across all HCNs [132]. These findings highlight the potential clinical importance of apparently benign HSV infection as a new factor in risk stratification for cancer of the lips, mouth and pharynx.

Other herpesviruses, such as cytomegalovirus (CMV), have been examined for their possible involvement in head and neck cancers (HNCs). Although the direct oncogenic roles of these viruses remain ambiguous, CMV and related viruses might play a part in cancer progression through mechanisms like chronic inflammation, immune modulation and interactions with other oncogenic elements. Typically not classified as oncogenic, CMV has nonetheless been associated with various cancers and has been the subject of clinical trials investigating its potential anti-tumor effects, particularly in relation to CMV-specific cytotoxic T cells and dendritic cell vaccines. Recently, Trivic et al. [133] conducted a worldwide study assessing the relationship between head and neck tumors and human CMV infection. Their 73-country study revealed a protective effect against malignancies of the salivary glands and lip/oral region, as well as a pro-oncogenic connection with nasopharyngeal carcinoma. However, when other variables associated with thyroid neoplasia and hypopharyngeal malignancies were taken into consideration, this protective effect vanished. There was no discernible link between CMV and laryngeal carcinoma. These results imply that CMV might have tissue-specific influences that could guide future treatment approaches for certain head and neck cancers, highlighting the necessity for additional studies to confirm these results and clarify the underlying mechanisms. It is yet unknown how herpesviruses other than HHV-1 contribute to head and neck malignancies. For instance, infections with HSV-1/HSV-2 have not been significantly associated with head and neck malignancies, while HHV-2 (HSV-2) has not been significantly associated with oral cancer. HHV-3 (Varicella-zoster virus) has been linked to an increased risk of cancer in people who have herpes zoster, despite the fact that it has not been proven to be a carcinogen. Although conclusive evidence is currently missing, salivary gland-resident HHV-6 and HHV-7 may have tumorigenic properties and the ability to activate other viruses, indicating a possible role in oral carcinogenesis. These results are examined in detail in the review of Wołacewicz et al. [134].

The ongoing investigation of these viruses in head and neck cancers (HNCs) shows potential for enhancing diagnostic, preventive and therapeutic strategies, which could ultimately lead to improved patient outcomes and quality of life.

4.5 Oncogenic impact of hepatitis viruses in HNCs

Hepatitis B (HBV) and C (HCV) are well-recognized carcinogens, particularly linked to non-Hodgkin lymphoma [135] and hepatocellular carcinoma [88]. Additionally, their role in increasing the risk of cancers beyond the liver is gaining acknowledgment. There is a growing interest in studying how hepatitis virus infections contribute to the development of HNCs [136, 137].

The genes for essential proteins required for HBV's viral activity, including surface antigens, core proteins, viral DNA polymerase and replication proteins, are found in this partly double-stranded DNA virus. Similar to EBV, HBV is dual-tropic, meaning it may infect hepatocytes as well as naive B cells. A DNA polymerase with reverse transcriptase activity promotes the transcription of viral RNA when the HBV genome enters the host cell and moves into the nucleus [138].

The genome of HCV, a positive-sense single-stranded RNA virus, encodes envelope glycoproteins and structural proteins. Hepatocytes, salivary gland cells and naive B cells are all infected by HCV, which has tritropic characteristics. HCV disrupts cell cycle control and inhibits apoptosis after infecting host cells, activating signaling pathways that support malignancy [139]. It is unclear exactly how HCV causes head and neck cancer, but it is comparable to HPV infection. By selectively breaking down proteins like p53 and Rb, HCV proteins like NS3 and NS5A interfere with the regulation of the cell cycle [140].

A retrospective case-control research was carried out by Donà et al. [141] to look at the connection between HNSCC and chronic hepatitis B and C infection. These findings highlight the need for more study to establish causality and the potential advantage of early discovery in enhancing patient outcomes by demonstrating an assertive relationship between chronic hepatitis B and C infection and HNSCC. Consistent results have been reported in Asian populations by Nayyar et al. in an Indian population [142] and Komori et al. in a Japanese population [143]. In order to investigate the relationship between HNC and positive hepatitis B core antibody (HBc), a sign of prior HBV infection, Komori conducted a retrospective case-control research. Positive HBc antibodies were found to be significantly associated with an elevated risk of HNC in the study, which included data from 495 non-HNC patients and 512 HNC patients treated between 2008 and 2017. Significant risk factors for HNC have also been shown to include smoking and a history of cancer [143]. These findings highlight the need for more research on the underlying biological mechanisms and suggest that HBV infection may contribute to the development of HNC in the Japanese population, despite limitations such selection bias and missing data on alcohol intake.

In contrast, a study conducted 12 years ago by Su et al. [144] discovered that a persistent HCV infection raises the risk of oral cancer by a large margin. Using Taiwanese national cohort data, scientists discovered that patients with HCV had a 2.28-fold increased risk of developing oral cancer in comparison to those who were not infected with the virus. HCV mono-infection was linked to a 90% increased risk of oral cancer after controlling for demographic variables, especially in persons between the ages of 40 and 49. On the other hand, the risk of oral cancer was not substantially correlated with either HBV mono-infection or HBV/HCV co-infection. Furthermore, Borsetto et al.'s meta-analysis [145] compiled data from eight observational studies and showed a strong correlation between a chronic HCV infection and a higher risk of HNSCC. Their conclusions showed that HCV-infected individuals have an increased hazard ratio for oral, oropharyngeal and laryngeal cancers. These findings demonstrate the significance of early invigilation for HNSCC in patients with chronic HCV infection and imply that HCV screening should be taken into account in the clinical management of HNSCC, even though a correlation with hypopharyngeal cancer has been proposed but was not statistically significant due to insufficient data. In order to investigate HBV and HCV infection, Hung et al. [146] carried out a case-control research with 5603 HNC patients and 16,809 matched controls. They found that the prevalence of HBV in HNC cases (9.0%) was higher than that in controls (7.6%). Alike, the prevalence of HCV was increased in HNC cases. In particular, the probability of HCV infection was significantly higher in patients with middle pharyngeal cancer compared to controls.

According to a meta-analysis conducted by Tan et al. [147], there is a significant positive correlation between HBV infection and HNC. HBV infection was linked to an increased incidence of HNC, according to their findings, which were based on a thorough analysis of 13 studies involving 58,006 individuals with HNC. Additional subgroup analyses revealed noteworthy correlations with nasopharyngeal carcinoma and mouth cancer. The extremely intriguing perspective of how HBV infection impacts survival in patients with HNSCC was investigated by Lai et al. [148]. They therefore discovered that HBV-positive subjects (12.3% of the population) had a greater incidence of liver cirrhosis and baseline hepatic dysfunction in their analysis of 1015 patients. HBV-positive patients exhibited a much worse 5-year overall and progression-free survival, even if their later rates of liver dysfunction were comparable. All of these findings point to the intricate relationship between HBV and HNSCC outcomes, which calls for specialized treatment strategies. New research continuously demonstrates a strong and intricate link between HBV and HCV infections and a higher chance of developing different kinds of HNC, especially oropharyngeal cancer. However, more investigation is required to clarify the underlying mechanisms causing these relationships and to settle any contradictory findings.

4.6 Merkel cell polyomavirus and its involvement in HNCs

Numerous ongoing investigations are attempting to clarify the function of human polyomaviruses, such MCPV, in the pathophysiology of HNCs, however this role has not been proved. Merkel cell carcinoma, an uncommon and aggressive neuroendocrine skin cancer, is linked to MCPV. But it has also been linked to the emergence of HNCs, especially pharyngeal and oral cancers. Similar to EBV infection, MCPV infection can linger in healthy individuals' skin and is frequently asymptomatic in childhood [149]. Mohebbi et al. [150] looked into MCPV in Iranian patients with HNSCC. They analyzed 50 biopsy specimens from HNSCC and discovered MCPV DNA in 16.0% of cases, with a greater viral burden in stage III tumors. The findings illustrated the need for more investigation by showing that MCPV infection may only impact a portion of HNSCC cases. In a different investigation, MCPV was found in 12.5% of the HNSCCs examined in Chilean patients by Muñoz et al. [151]. BK human polyomavirus (BKPV) and JC human polyomavirus (JCPV), on the other hand, were not frequently detected. Significantly, MCPV was not found in the mouthbrushes of those without cancer, indicating that MCPV may be particularly linked to HNSCCs. Both malignant and non-cancerous oral lesions may be affected by MCPV. In a study carried out in Northern Iran, Estalkhi et al. [152] compared the prevalence of MCPV in 114 oral cavity biopsies between non-cancerous diseases [oral lichen planus (OLP) and oral irritation fibroma (OIF)] and malignant lesions (OSCC, dysplasia). Twenty percent of OSCC samples, 21 percent of dysplasia samples, 21 percent of OLP samples and 36 percent of OIF samples had MCPV DNA. These findings imply that additional study is necessary to completely comprehend how MCPV contributes to the development of HNCs.

4.7 Intricacies of co-infections in HNCs

The carcinogenic potential of viruses in the head and neck region can be impacted by co-infections with other pathogens, which can exacerbate the progression of cancer through a variety of mechanisms. These interactions frequently result in immunosuppression, persistent inflammation and synergistic cellular damage, creating more conducive conditions for the spread of cancer. Importantly, HIV-induced immunosuppression increases the incidence of HPV-associated malignancies at various anatomical locations, including HNCs [153]. These tumors tend to act more aggressively and show up at more advanced stages. Due to their weakened immune systems, which make it more difficult to effectively eradicate the virus, people with HIV are more prone to experience persistent HPV infections. The likelihood of oncogenic mutations and the development of cancer is increased by this persistence. Additionally, although antiretroviral medication improves overall immune function, it does not completely eliminate the increased risk of cancer, which emphasizes the need for careful cancer screening and prolepsis strategies in these individuals [86].

Additionally, Salahuddin et al. [154] discovered in their research that individuals with HIV (PWH) and HNC have much worse clinical outcomes than patients without the virus. A worse overall survival was independently predicted by HIV, with PWH having a median survival of 39.1 months compared to 100.8 months for patients without the virus. This difference was most noticeable in OPSCC linked to HPV and early-stage malignancies. Additionally, PWH neoplasms exhibited reduced PD-L1 expression and CD8 T-cell infiltration, both of which are linked to improved outcomes. It is essential to conduct additional research on HIV-related HNC and develop tailored treatment plans for this population.

An inflammatory milieu created by persistent bacterial infections can promote viral persistence and carcinogenesis [155]. One common example is *Helicobacter pylori*, which has a long history of being linked to gastric cancer [156]. Oncogenesis may be accelerated by the synergistic interactions of several bacteria species present in the oral cavity. Notably, a higher incidence of oral and oropharyngeal malignancies has been linked to chronic periodontitis, a common oral infection. By disrupting normal cellular homeostasis and impairing local immune responses, the persistent inflammation caused by periodontitis creates an environment that is favorable for oncogenic viruses [157]. Additionally, periodontitis causes the release of cytokines and free radicals, which are processes linked to carcinogenic and metastatic activity [158]. Furthermore, long-term bacterial infections might encourage the Epithelial–Mesenchymal Transition (EMT), a process that gives epithelial cells mesenchymal characteristics and enhances their capacity for migration and invasion. One of the most important pillars of cancer metastasis is EMT. Signaling pathways including STAT3 and NF-κB, which are known to have roles in inflammation and cancer formation, can also be activated by bacterial infections and the associated inflammatory responses [159]. Tactical dental examinations, prompt treatment of periodontal diseases and good tooth hygiene are crucial in reducing these risks.

The risk of cancer may also be increased by co-infection with multiple carcinogenic viruses. Various studies have reported co-infection with HPV and EBV in HNC [160, 161]. Through molecular interactions, these viruses enhance one another's capacity to cause cancer. HPV's capacity to evade immune detection and stimulate cell proliferation may be enhanced by EBV's function in regulating the immune response and creating an inflammatory milieu. Interactions between these viruses may result in inferior clinical outcomes and more aggressive tumor morphologies [162]. With incidences ranging from 15 to 20% globally and higher rates (25–70%) in squamous cell carcinomas of the tonsils and base of the tongue, EBV and HPV co-infection significantly affect oropharyngeal carcinomas [163]. Co-infection *in vitro* has been demonstrated to advance viral replication and influence viral cycle dynamics. HPV may influence EBV latency, whereas EBV delays epithelial development and encourages invasiveness, especially in cells that express the HPV-16 E6 and E7 oncogenes [117]. Their cooperative involvement in cancer progression was highlighted by a study conducted in Bosnia that found a 34.7% co-infection rate in HNSCC tissues, which was substantially linked with advanced illness [164]. To fully clarify the concrete contribution of EBV to HPV-positive oropharyngeal cancer, more investigation is required.

Oncogenic viruses in HNSCC in Romanian patients were examined by Ursu et al. [165]. After testing 26 tumors for 67 viral components, they discovered that 88.5% of them tested positive for one or more viruses, particularly HPV. According to their research, EBV-1, HHV-7 and MCPV were commonly found, and herpes and polyomaviruses were much more prevalent in HPV-negative patients. This suggests that these viruses may have a role in the development of these tumors.

Mulder et al. [166] investigated the presence of HPV, EBV and MCPV in HNSCC of non-smokers and non-drinkers (NSND). They discovered EBV in three oropharyngeal tumors and HPV in all oropharyngeal malignancies and one oral tumor. They were unable to identify MCPV, though. Overall survival and 5-year disease-free survival were not significantly impacted by HPV or EBV positive. More research on virus-negative tumors for targeted therapy is desperately needed, as the roles of HPV and EBV, in particular HNSCC subtypes between NSND, are limited in terms of survival outcomes.

In a cohort of 78 patients, Schindele et al. used advanced molecular techniques to analyze the presence of EBV, CMV and human adenovirus (HAdV). The outcomes displayed that EBV was present in 33% of tumor samples and CMV and HAdV were less frequent, showing a mutable prevalence of these viruses in LSCC. The fingering of high-risk HPV-16 in 9% of samples emphasizes its potential role, but overexpression of p16 was more commonly remarked in 14% of cases [167].

The comprehension and treatment of those interactions is very important in developing a comprehensive strategy to contend HNC. Targeting inflammatory pathways and managing chronic infections may help decrease the growth and progression of HNC.

5. Conclusions

The intricate viral environment in HNC is essential to the development and spread of the malignancy. Carcinogenesis is caused by interactions between viruses and other genetic and environmental variables as well as by a lengthy latency period (**Figure 10**). Viruses can evade immune monitoring, interfere with regular cell cycle

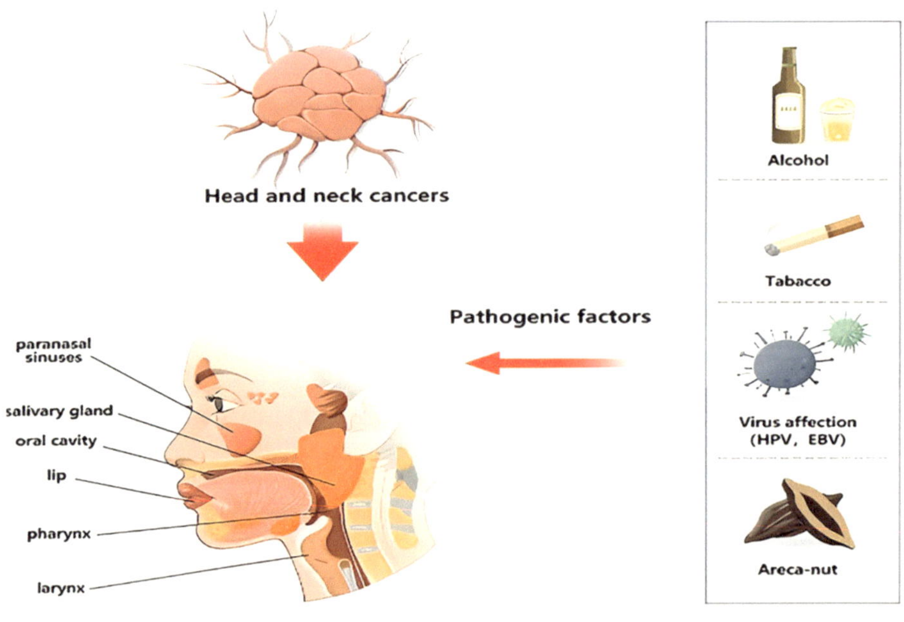

Figure 10.
Illustration depicting the multifactorial pathogenesis of HNC, giving emphasis to the role of carcinogenic viruses in combination with environmental factors [168].

regulation and integrate into the host's DNA. These processes lead to malignant transformation and tumor growth when paired with exposure to toxins and genetic predispositions. Novel treatments and diagnostic biomarkers may result from recent developments in the identification of viral proteins and their interactions with host cells. Therapeutic results could be greatly enhanced by customized strategies catered to the unique viral profile of HNC. To completely understand these mechanisms and facilitate the creation of efficient management plans for virus-related HNC, more research is necessary. We may learn more about the effects of viruses on human health in the post-COVID age if studies find additional viruses that have the potential to cause cancer or modify the immune system.

Author details

Eleni Litsou
University Hospital of Ioannina, Greece

*Address all correspondence to: elenilitsou@gmail.com

References

[1] Kamiński B. Lymphomas of the head-and-neck region. Journal of Cancer Research and Therapeutics. 2021;**17**(6):1347-1350. DOI: 10.4103/jcrt.JCRT_213_20

[2] Bhat GR, Hyole RG, Li J. Head and neck cancer: Current challenges and future perspectives. Advances in Cancer Research. 2021;**152**:67-102. DOI: 10.1016/bs.acr.2021.05.002. Epub 2021 Jun 16

[3] Ferlay J, Shin HR, Bray F, Forman D, Mathers C, Parkin DM. Estimates of worldwide burden of cancer in 2008: GLOBOCAN 2008. International Journal of Cancer. 2010;**127**(12):2893-2917. DOI: 10.1002/ijc.25516

[4] Adamopoulos G. Otolaryngology and Head and Neck Surgery: General Knowledge, Head and Neck Cancer. 2nd ed. Athens: Paschalidis Medical Publications; 2006. p. 1266

[5] Li Q, Tie Y, Alu A, Ma X, Shi H. Targeted therapy for head and neck cancer: Signaling pathways and clinical studies. Signal Transduction and Targeted Therapy. 2023;**8**(1):31. DOI: 10.1038/s41392-022-01297-0

[6] Payaradka R, Ramesh PS, Vyas R, Patil P, Rajendra VK, Kumar M, et al. Oncogenic viruses as etiological risk factors for head and neck cancers: An overview on prevalence, mechanism of infection and clinical relevance. Archives of Oral Biology. 2022;**143**:105526. DOI: 10.1016/j.archoralbio.2022.105526. Epub 2022 Aug 20

[7] Moore PS, Chang Y. Why do viruses cause cancer? Highlights of the first century of human tumour virology. Nature Reviews. Cancer. 2010;**10**(12):878-889. DOI: 10.1038/nrc2961. Epub 2010 Nov 24

[8] Samara P, Athanasopoulos M, Mastronikolis S, Kyrodimos E, Athanasopoulos I, Mastronikolis NS. The role of oncogenic viruses in head and neck cancers: Epidemiology, pathogenesis, and advancements in detection methods. Microorganisms. 2024;**12**(7):1482. DOI: 10.3390/microorganisms12071482

[9] Tempera I, Lieberman PM. Oncogenic viruses as entropic drivers of cancer evolution. Frontiers in Virology. 2021;**1**:753366. DOI: 10.3389/fviro.2021.753366. Epub 2021 Nov 15

[10] Narisawa-Saito M, Kiyono T. Basic mechanisms of high-risk human papillomavirus-induced carcinogenesis: Roles of E6 and E7 proteins. Cancer Science. 2007;**98**(10):1505-1511. DOI: 10.1111/j.1349-7006.2007.00546.x. Epub 2007 Jul 23

[11] Ndon S, Singh A, Ha PK, Aswani J, Chan JY, Xu MJ. Human papillomavirus-associated oropharyngeal cancer: Global epidemiology and public policy implications. Cancers (Basel). 2023;**15**(16):4080. DOI: 10.3390/cancers15164080

[12] Prabhu SR, Wilson DF. Evidence of Epstein-Barr virus association with head and neck cancers: A review. Journal of the Canadian Dental Association. 2016;**82**:g2. Available from: https://jcda.ca/g2

[13] Leemans CR, Snijders PJF, Brakenhoff RH. The molecular landscape of head and neck cancer. Nature Reviews. Cancer. 2018;**18**(5):269-282. DOI: 10.1038/nrc.2018.11. Epub 2018 Mar 2. Erratum in: Nat Rev Cancer. 2018 Oct;18(10):662. doi: 10.1038/s41568-018-0057-9

[14] Swiecicki PL, Brennan JR, Mierzwa M, Spector ME, Brenner JC. Head and neck squamous cell carcinoma detection and surveillance: Advances of liquid biomarkers. The Laryngoscope. 2019;**129**(8):1836-1843. DOI: 10.1002/lary.27725. Epub 2018 Dec 20

[15] Mukherjee S, Fischbein NJ, Baugnon KL, Policeni BA, Raghavan P. Contemporary imaging and reporting strategies for head and neck cancer: MRI, FDG PET/MRI, NI-RADS, and carcinoma of unknown primary-AJR expert panel narrative review. AJR. American Journal of Roentgenology. 2023;**220**(2):160-172. DOI: 10.2214/AJR.22.28120. Epub 2022 Sep 7

[16] Carcinogenesis [Internet]. 2020 [cited 2024 Dec 11]. Available from: https://med.libretexts.org/@go/page/2161

[17] Krikelis D. Detection of the HPV16 E7 Oncogene in Epithelial Carcinomas, Correlation with Hypermethylation in the p16 Gene Promoter. Thessaloniki: Aristotle University of Thessaloniki; 2009

[18] Panagi A. Oncogenes and tumor suppressor genes. In: Clinical Oncology. Volume a, General Part. EEPOE: Athens; 2007. pp. 139-155

[19] Brinkman BM, Wong DT. Disease mechanism and biomarkers of oral squamous cell carcinoma. Current Opinion in Oncology. 2006;**18**(3):228-233. DOI: 10.1097/01.cco.0000219250.15041.f8

[20] Hanahan D, Weinberg RA. The hallmarks of cancer. Cell. 2000;**100**(1):57-70. DOI: 10.1016/s0092-8674(00)81683-9

[21] Negrini S, Gorgoulis VG, Halazonetis TD. Genomic instability–an evolving hallmark of cancer. Nature Reviews. Molecular Cell Biology. 2010;**11**(3):220-228. DOI: 10.1038/nrm2858

[22] Farber E. The multistep nature of cancer development. Cancer Research. 1984;**44**(10):4217-4223. Available from: https://pubmed.ncbi.nlm.nih.gov/6467183/

[23] Bedi GC, Westra WH, Gabrielson E, Koch W, Sidransky D. Multiple head and neck tumors: Evidence for a common clonal origin. Cancer Research. 1996;**56**(11):2484-2487. Available from: https://pubmed.ncbi.nlm.nih.gov/8653681/

[24] Slaughter DP, Southwick HW, Smejkal W. Field cancerization in oral stratified squamous epithelium; clinical implications of multicentric origin. Cancer. 1953;**6**(5):963-968. DOI: 10.1002/1097-0142(195309)6:5<963::aid-cncr2820060515>3.0.co;2-q

[25] Leemans CR, Braakhuis BJ, Brakenhoff RH. The molecular biology of head and neck cancer. Nature Reviews. Cancer. 2011;**11**(1):9-22. DOI: 10.1038/nrc2982. Epub 2010 Dec 16

[26] Choi S, Myers JN. Molecular pathogenesis of oral squamous cell carcinoma: Implications for therapy. Journal of Dental Research. 2008;**87**(1):14-32. DOI: 10.1177/154405910808700104. Erratum in: J Dent Res. 2008 Feb; 87(2):191

[27] Perez-Ordoñez B, Beauchemin M, Jordan RC. Molecular biology of squamous cell carcinoma of the head and neck. Journal of Clinical Pathology. 2006;**59**(5):445-453. DOI: 10.1136/jcp.2003.007641

[28] Cardesa A, Nadal A. Carcinoma of the head and neck in the HPV era. Acta

Dermatovenerologica Alpina, Panonica et Adriatica. 2011;**20**(3):161-173. Available from: https://pubmed.ncbi.nlm.nih.gov/22131117/

[29] Choe MS, Zhang X, Shin HJ, Shin DM, Chen ZG. Interaction between epidermal growth factor receptor- and cyclooxygenase 2-mediated pathways and its implications for the chemoprevention of head and neck cancer. Molecular Cancer Therapeutics. 2005;**4**(9):1448-1455. DOI: 10.1158/1535-7163.MCT-04-0251

[30] Zur HH. Oncogenic DNA viruses. Oncogene. 2001;**20**(54):7820-7823. DOI: 10.1038/sj.onc.1204958

[31] Parsonnet J. In: Parsonnet J, editor. Microbes and Malignancy. New York: Oxford Univ. Press; 1999. pp. 3-18

[32] Steele C, Cowsert LM, Shillitoe EJ. Effects of human papillomavirus type 18-specific antisense oligonucleotides on the transformed phenotype of human carcinoma cell lines. Cancer Research. 1993;**53**(Suppl. 10):2330-2337. Available from: https://pubmed.ncbi.nlm.nih.gov/7683572/

[33] Tan TM, Ting RC. In vitro and in vivo inhibition of human papillomavirus type 16 E6 and E7 genes. Cancer Research. 1995;**55**:4599-4605. Available from: https://pubmed.ncbi.nlm.nih.gov/7553636/

[34] Goodwin EC, DiMaio D. Repression of human papillomavirus oncogenes in HeLa cervical carcinoma cells causes the orderly reactivation of dormant tumor suppressor pathways. Proceedings of the National Academy of Sciences of the United States of America. 2000;**97**(23):12513-12518. DOI: 10.1073/pnas.97.23.12513

[35] Wies E, Mori Y, Hahn A, Kremmer E, Stürzl M, Fleckenstein B, et al. The viral interferon-regulatory factor-3 is required for the survival of KSHV-infected primary effusion lymphoma cells. Blood. 2008;**111**(1):320-327. DOI: 10.1182/blood-2007-05-092288. Epub 2007 Sep 21

[36] Houben R, Shuda M, Weinkam R, Schrama D, Feng H, Chang Y, et al. Merkel cell polyomavirus-infected Merkel cell carcinoma cells require expression of viral T antigens. Journal of Virology. 2010;**84**(14):7064-7072. DOI: 10.1128/JVI.02400-09. Epub 2010 May 5

[37] Godfrey A, Anderson J, Papanastasiou A, Takeuchi Y, Boshoff C. Inhibiting primary effusion lymphoma by lentiviral vectors encoding short hairpin RNA. Blood. 2005;**105**(6):2510-2518. DOI: 10.1182/blood-2004-08-3052. Epub 2004 Nov 30

[38] Dirmeier U, Hoffmann R, Kilger E, Schultheiss U, Briseño C, Gires O, et al. Latent membrane protein 1 of Epstein-Barr virus coordinately regulates proliferation with control of apoptosis. Oncogene. 2005;**24**(10):1711-1717. DOI: 10.1038/sj.onc.1208367

[39] Cotran RS, Kumar V, Collins T. Robbins Pathologic Basis of Disease. 6th ed. Philadelphia, PA: W.B. Saunders Company; 1999. pp. 311-315, 340-341, 888-889

[40] Levine AJ. The common mechanisms of transformation by the small DNA tumor viruses: The inactivation of tumor suppressor gene products: p53. Virology. 2009;**384**(2):285-293. DOI: 10.1016/j.virol.2008.09.034. Epub 2008 Dec 11

[41] Oh ST, Kyo S, Laimins LA. Telomerase activation by human papillomavirus type 16 E6 protein: Induction of human telomerase reverse transcriptase expression through Myc and GC-rich Sp1 binding sites. Journal

of Virology. 2001;**75**(12):5559-5566. DOI: 10.1128/JVI.75.12.5559-5566.2001

[42] Verma SC, Borah S, Robertson ES. Latency-associated nuclear antigen of Kaposi's sarcoma-associated herpesvirus up-regulates transcription of human telomerase reverse transcriptase promoter through interaction with transcription factor Sp1. Journal of Virology. 2004;**78**(19):10348-10359. DOI: 10.1128/JVI.78.19.10348-10359.2004

[43] Terrin L, Dal Col J, Rampazzo E, Zancai P, Pedrotti M, Ammirabile G, et al. Latent membrane protein 1 of Epstein-Barr virus activates the hTERT promoter and enhances telomerase activity in B lymphocytes. Journal of Virology. 2008;**82**(20):10175-10187. DOI: 10.1128/JVI.00321-08. Epub 2008 Aug 6

[44] Buchkovich NJ, Yu Y, Zampieri CA, Alwine JC. The TORrid affairs of viruses: Effects of mammalian DNA viruses on the PI3K-Akt-mTOR signalling pathway. Nature Reviews. Microbiology. 2008;**6**(4):266-275. DOI: 10.1038/nrmicro1855. Epub 2008 Mar 3

[45] Liu L, Eby MT, Rathore N, Sinha SK, Kumar A, Chaudhary PM. The human herpes virus 8-encoded viral FLICE inhibitory protein physically associates with and persistently activates the Ikappa B kinase complex. The Journal of Biological Chemistry. 2002;**277**(16):13745-13751. DOI: 10.1074/jbc.M110480200. Epub 2002 Feb 5

[46] Fujimuro M, Wu FY, ApRhys C, Kajumbula H, Young DB, Hayward GS, et al. A novel viral mechanism for dysregulation of beta-catenin in Kaposi's sarcoma-associated herpesvirus latency. Nature Medicine. 2003;**9**(3):300-306. DOI: 10.1038/nm829. Epub 2003 Feb 18

[47] Moore PS, Chang Y. Antiviral activity of tumor-suppressor pathways: Clues from molecular piracy by KSHV. Trends in Genetics. 1998;**14**(4):144-150. DOI: 10.1016/s0168-9525(98)01408-5

[48] Nagpal JK, Das BR. Oral cancer: Reviewing the present understanding of its molecular mechanism and exploring the future directions for its effective management. Oral Oncology. 2003;**39**(3):213-221. DOI: 10.1016/s1368-8375(02)00162-8

[49] Zourboulis B, Solakidis S. The role of the tumor suppressor protein p53 in cancer. Oncology Update. 2003;**5**:98-103

[50] Popović B, Jekić B, Novaković I, Luković L, Konstantinović V, Babić M, et al. Cancer genes alterations and HPV infection in oral squamous cell carcinoma. International Journal of Oral and Maxillofacial Surgery. 2010;**39**(9):909-915. DOI: 10.1016/j.ijom.2010.05.007. Epub 2010 Jun 26

[51] Pérez-Sayáns M, Somoza-Martín JM, Barros-Angueira F, Reboiras-López MD, Gándara Rey JM, García-García A. Genetic and molecular alterations associated with oral squamous cell cancer (review). Oncology Reports. 2009;**22**(6):1277-1282. DOI: 10.3892/or_00000565

[52] Supić G, Kozomara R, Branković-Magić M, Jović N, Magić Z. Gene hypermethylation in tumor tissue of advanced oral squamous cell carcinoma patients. Oral Oncology. 2009;**45**(12):1051-1057. DOI: 10.1016/j.oraloncology.2009.07.007. Epub 2009 Aug 8

[53] Campo-Trapero J, Cano-Sánchez J, Palacios-Sánchez B, Sánchez-Gutierrez JJ, González-Moles MA, Bascones-Martínez A. Update on molecular pathology in oral cancer and precancer. Anticancer Research. 2008;**28**(2B):1197-1205. Available

from: https://pubmed.ncbi.nlm.nih.gov/18505056/

[54] Westra WH. The changing face of head and neck cancer in the 21st century: The impact of HPV on the epidemiology and pathology of oral cancer. Head and Neck Pathology. 2009;**3**(1):78-81. DOI: 10.1007/s12105-009-0100-y. Epub 2009 Feb 24

[55] MacLennan SA, Marra MA. Oncogenic viruses and the Epigenome: How viruses hijack epigenetic mechanisms to drive cancer. International Journal of Molecular Sciences. 2023;**24**(11):9543. DOI: 10.3390/ijms24119543

[56] Coffin JM, Hughes SH, Varmus HE, editors. Retroviruses. Cold Spring Harbor (NY): Cold Spring Harbor Laboratory Press; 1997. PMID: 21433340. Bookshelf ID: NBK19376

[57] Parsonnet J. *Helicobacter* and gastric adenocarcinoma. In: Parsonnet J, editor. Microbes and Malignancy: Infection as a Cause of Human Cancers. New York, NY: Oxford University Press; 1999. pp. 372-408

[58] Levine AJ. The tumor suppressor genes. Annual Review of Biochemistry. 1993;**62**:623-651. DOI: 10.1146/annurev.bi.62.070193.003203

[59] Rosenberg N, Jolicoeur P. In: Coffin J, Hughes S, Varmus HE, editors. Retrovirus Pathogenesis, Retroviruses. Cold Spring Harbor, NY: Cold Spring Harbor Laboratory Press; 1997. pp. 475-585

[60] Kung HJ, Boerkoel C, Carter TH. Retroviral mutagenesis of cellular oncogenes: A review with insights into the mechanisms of insertional activation. Current Topics in Microbiology and Immunology. 1991;**171**:1-25. DOI: 10.1007/978-3-642-76524-7_1

[61] Fourel G, Trepo C, Bougueleret L, Henglein B, Ponzetto A, Tiollais P, et al. Frequent activation of N-myc genes by hepadnavirus insertion in woodchuck liver tumours. Nature. 1990;**347**(6290):294-298. DOI: 10.1038/347294a0

[62] Levinson W. Review of Medical Microbiology and Immunology. 13th ed. California, San Francisco: Smartbook™ McGraw Hill Professional; 2014. ISBN: 007181812X, 9780071818124

[63] Thelander L, Reichard P. Reduction of ribonucleotides. Annual Review of Biochemistry. 1979;**48**:133-158. DOI: 10.1146/annurev.bi.48.070179.001025

[64] Nevins JR, Vogt PK. Cell transformation by viruses. In: Fields BN, Knipe DM, Howley PM, editors. Fields Virology. 3rd ed. NewYork: Raven Press, Ltd.; 1996. pp. 301-343

[65] Peters G, Vousden KH, editors. Oncogenes and Tumour Suppressors. Oxford: IRL Press at Oxford University Press; 1997

[66] Lane DP, Crawford LV. T antigen is bound to a host protein in SV40-transformed cells. Nature. 1979;**278**(5701):261-263. DOI: 10.1038/278261a0

[67] Finlay CA, Hinds PW, Levine AJ. The p53 proto-oncogene can act as a suppressor of transformation. Cell. 1989;**57**(7):1083-1093. DOI: 10.1016/0092-8674(89)90045-7

[68] Ghoreshi ZA, Molaei HR, Arefinia N. The role of DNA viruses in human cancer. Cancer Informatics. 2023;**22**:11769351231208757. DOI: 10.1177/11769351231154186

[69] Amundson SA, Myers TG, Fornace AJ Jr. Roles for p53 in growth arrest and apoptosis: Putting on the brakes after genotoxic stress. Oncogene. 1998;**17**(25):3287-3299. DOI: 10.1038/sj.onc.1202576

[70] Sukumar S, Notario V, Martin-Zanca D, Barbacid M. Induction of mammary carcinomas in rats by nitroso-methylurea involves malignant activation of H-ras-1 locus by single point mutations. Nature. 1983;**306**(5944):658-661. DOI: 10.1038/306658a0

[71] Look AT. Oncogenic transcription factors in the human acute leukemias. Science. 1997;**278**(5340):1059-1064. DOI: 10.1126/science.278.5340.1059

[72] Kew MC. Hepatocellular carcinoma with and without cirrhosis.A comparison in southern African blacks. Gastroenterology. 1989;**97**(1):136-139. DOI: 10.1016/0016-5085(89)91426-1

[73] Howley PM. Polyomavirinae: The viruses and their replication. In: Fields BC, Knipe DM, Howley PM, editors. Fields Virology. Vol. 1996. Philadelphia: Lippincott-Raven Publishers; 1997-2043. pp. 947-978

[74] de Sanjosé S, Brotons M, Pavón MA. The natural history of human papillomavirus infection. Best Practice & Research. Clinical Obstetrics & Gynaecology. 2018;**47**:2-13. DOI: 10.1016/j.bpobgyn.2017.08.015. Epub 2017 Sep 6

[75] Scheurer ME, Tortolero-Luna G, Adler-Storthz K. Human papillomavirus infection: Biology, epidemiology, and prevention. International Journal of Gynecological Cancer. 2005;**15**(5):727-746. DOI: 10.1111/j.1525-1438.2005.00246.x

[76] Kobayashi K, Hisamatsu K, Suzui N, Hara A, Tomita H, Miyazaki T. A review of HPV-related head and neck cancer. Journal of Clinical Medicine. 2018;**7**(9):241. DOI: 10.3390/jcm7090241

[77] Doorbar J. Model systems of human papillomavirus-associated disease. The Journal of Pathology. 2016;**238**(2):166-179. DOI: 10.1002/path.4656. Epub 2015 Dec 10

[78] Kajitani N, Satsuka A, Kawate A, Sakai H. Productive lifecycle of human papillomaviruses that depends upon squamous epithelial differentiation. Frontiers in Microbiology. 2012;**3**:152. DOI: 10.3389/fmicb.2012.00152

[79] Fernandes JV, Galvão de Araújo JM, de Medeiros Fernandes T. Biology and natural history of human papillomavirus infection. Open access. Journal of Clinical Trials. 2013;**5**:1-12

[80] Frazer I. Prevention of cervical cancer through papillomavirus vaccination. Nature Reviews. Immunology. 2004;**4**:46-55. DOI: 10.1038/nri1260

[81] Moody CA, Laimins LA. Human papillomavirus oncoproteins: Pathways to transformation. Nature Reviews. Cancer. 2010;**10**(8):550-560. DOI: 10.1038/nrc2886. Epub 2010 Jul 1

[82] Burd EM. Human papillomavirus and cervical cancer. Clinical Microbiology Reviews. 2003;**16**(1):1-17. DOI: 10.1128/CMR.16.1.1-17.2003

[83] Chaturvedi AK, Engels EA, Pfeiffer RM, Hernandez BY, Xiao W, Kim E, et al. Human papillomavirus and rising oropharyngeal cancer incidence in the United States. Journal of Clinical Oncology. 2011;**29**(32):4294-4301. DOI: 10.1200/JCO.2011.36.4596. Epub 2011 Oct 3

[84] Gillison ML, Koch WM, Capone RB, Spafford M, Westra WH, Wu L, et al.

Evidence for a causal association between human papillomavirus and a subset of head and neck cancers. Journal of the National Cancer Institute. 2000;**92**(9):709-720. DOI: 10.1093/jnci/92.9.709

[85] Fakhry C, Westra WH, Li S, Cmelak A, Ridge JA, Pinto H, et al. Improved survival of patients with human papillomavirus-positive head and neck squamous cell carcinoma in a prospective clinical trial. Journal of the National Cancer Institute. 2008;**100**(4):261-269. DOI: 10.1093/jnci/djn011. Epub 2008 Feb 12

[86] Chaturvedi AK, Madeleine MM, Biggar RJ, Engels EA. Risk of human papillomavirus-associated cancers among persons with AIDS. Journal of the National Cancer Institute. 2009;**101**(16):1120-1130. DOI: 10.1093/jnci/djp205. Epub 2009 Jul 31

[87] Blomberg M, Nielsen A, Munk C, Kjaer SK. Trends in head and neck cancer incidence in Denmark, 1978-2007: Focus on human papillomavirus associated sites. International Journal of Cancer. 2011;**129**(3):733-741. DOI: 10.1002/ijc.25699. Epub 2010 Oct 26

[88] D'souza S, Lau KC, Coffin CS, Patel TR. Molecular mechanisms of viral hepatitis induced hepatocellular carcinoma. World Journal of Gastroenterology. 2020;**26**(38):5759-5783. DOI: 10.3748/wjg.v26.i38.5759

[89] Vinokurova S, Wentzensen N, Kraus I, Klaes R, Driesch C, Melsheimer P, et al. Type-dependent integration frequency of human papillomavirus genomes in cervical lesions. Cancer Research. 2008;**68**(1):307-313. DOI: 10.1158/0008-5472.CAN-07-2754

[90] Pinatti LM, Walline HM, Carey TE. Human papillomavirus genome integration and head and neck cancer. Journal of Dental Research. 2018;**97**(6):691-700. DOI: 10.1177/0022034517744213. Epub 2017 Dec 11

[91] Akagi K, Li J, Broutian TR, Padilla-Nash H, Xiao W, Jiang B, et al. Genome-wide analysis of HPV integration in human cancers reveals recurrent, focal genomic instability. Genome Research. 2014;**24**(2):185-199. DOI: 10.1101/gr.164806.113. Epub 2013 Nov 7

[92] Pai SI, Westra WH. Molecular pathology of head and neck cancer: Implications for diagnosis, prognosis, and treatment. Annual Review of Pathology. 2009;**4**:49-70. DOI: 10.1146/annurev.pathol.4.110807.092158

[93] Liberale C, Soloperto D, Marchioni A, Monzani D, Sacchetto L. Updates on larynx cancer: Risk factors and Oncogenesis. International Journal of Molecular Sciences. 2023;**24**(16):12913. DOI: 10.3390/ijms241612913

[94] Li X, Gao L, Li H, Gao J, Yang Y, Zhou F, et al. Human papillomavirus infection and laryngeal cancer risk: A systematic review and meta-analysis. The Journal of Infectious Diseases. 2013;**207**(3):479-488. DOI: 10.1093/infdis/jis698. Epub 2012 Nov 21

[95] Gama RR, Carvalho AL, Longatto Filho A, Scorsato AP, López RV, Rautava J, et al. Detection of human papillomavirus in laryngeal squamous cell carcinoma: Systematic review and meta-analysis. The Laryngoscope. 2016;**126**(4):885-893. DOI: 10.1002/lary.25738. Epub 2015 Nov 6

[96] Aaltonen LM, Rihkanen H, Vaheri A. Human papillomavirus in larynx. The Laryngoscope. 2002;**112**(4):700-707. DOI: 10.1097/00005537-200204000-00020

[97] Bosch FX, Muñoz N. The viral etiology of cervical cancer. Virus Research. 2002;**89**(2):183-190. DOI: 10.1016/s0168-1702(02)00187-9

[98] Erkul E, Yilmaz I, Narli G, Babayigit MA, Gungor A, Demirel D. The presence and prognostic significance of human papillomavirus in squamous cell carcinoma of the larynx. European Archives of Oto-Rhino-Laryngology. 2017 Jul;**274**(7):2921-2926. DOI: 10.1007/s00405-017-4573-0. Epub 2017 Apr 21

[99] Braakhuis BJ, Tabor MP, Leemans CR, van der Waal I, Snow GB, Brakenhoff RH. Second primary tumors and field cancerization in oral and oropharyngeal cancer: Molecular techniques provide new insights and definitions. Head & Neck. 2002;**24**(2):198-206. DOI: 10.1002/hed.10042

[100] Burkitt D. A children's cancer dependent on climatic factors. Nature. 1962;**194**:232-234. DOI: 10.1038/194232a0

[101] Epstein MA, Achong BG, Barr YM. Virus particles in cultured lymphoblasts from Burkitt's lymphoma. Lancet. 1964;**1**(7335):702-703. DOI: 10.1016/s0140-6736(64)91524-7

[102] Henle W, Diehl V, Kohn G, Zur Hausen H, Henle G. Herpes-type virus and chromosome marker in normal leukocytes after growth with irradiated Burkitt cells. Science. 1967;**157**(3792):1064-1065. DOI: 10.1126/science.157.3792.1064

[103] Cho Y, Ramer J, Rivailler P, Quink C, Garber RL, Beier DR, et al. An Epstein-Barr-related herpesvirus from marmoset lymphomas. Proceedings of the National Academy of Sciences of the United States of America. 2001;**98**(3):1224-1229. DOI: 10.1073/pnas.98.3.1224

[104] Chang Y, Cesarman E, Pessin MS, Lee F, Culpepper J, Knowles DM, et al. Identification of herpesvirus-like DNA sequences in AIDS-associated Kaposi's sarcoma. Science. 1994;**266**(5192):1865-1869. DOI: 10.1126/science.7997879

[105] Nilsson K, Klein G, Henle W, Henle G. The establishment of lymphoblastoid lines from adult and fetal human lymphoid tissue and its dependence on EBV. International Journal of Cancer. 1971;**8**(3):443-450. DOI: 10.1002/ijc.2910080312

[106] Gerber P, Lucas S, Nonoyama M, Perlin E, Goldstein LI. Oral excretion of Epstein-Barr virus by healthy subjects and patients with infectious mononucleosis. Lancet. 1972;**2**(7785):988-989. DOI: 10.1016/s0140-6736(72)92402-6

[107] Evans AS, Niederman JC, McCollum RW. Seroepidemiologic studies of infectious mononucleosis with EB virus. The New England Journal of Medicine. 1968;**279**(21):1121-1127. DOI: 10.1056/NEJM196811212792101

[108] Horwitz CA, Henle W, Henle G, Schapiro R, Borken S, Bundtzen R. Infectious mononucleosis in patients aged 40 to 72 years: Report of 27 cases, including 3 without heterophil-antibody responses. Medicine (Baltimore). 1983;**62**(4):256-262. DOI: 10.1097/00005792-198307000-00005

[109] Gerber P, Walsh JH, Rosenblum EN, Purcell RH. Association of EB-virus infection with the post-perfusion syndrome. Lancet. 1969;**1**(7595):593-595. DOI: 10.1016/s0140-6736(69)91532-3

[110] Damania B, Kenney SC, Raab-Traub N. Epstein-Barr virus: Biology and clinical disease. Cell.

2022;**185**(20):3652-3670. DOI: 10.1016/j.cell.2022.08.026. Epub 2022 Sep 15

[111] Bakkalci D, Jia Y, Winter JR, Lewis JE, Taylor GS, Stagg HR. Risk factors for Epstein Barr virus-associated cancers: A systematic review, critical appraisal, and mapping of the epidemiological evidence. Journal of Global Health. 2020;**10**(1):010405. DOI: 10.7189/jogh.10.010405

[112] Scott RS. Epstein-Barr virus: A master epigenetic manipulator. Current Opinion in Virology. 2017;**26**:74-80. DOI: 10.1016/j.coviro.2017.07.017. Epub 2017 Aug 4

[113] Longnecker R, Kieff E, Cohen JI. Epstein-Barr virus. In: Knipe DM, Howley PM, editors. Fields Virology. 6th ed. Vol. 2. Philadelphia, PA, USA: Lippincott Williams & Wilkins; 2013. pp. 1898-1959

[114] Liebowitz D, Kieff E. Epstein-Barr virus. In: Roizman B, Whitley RJ, Lopez C, editors. The Human Herpesvirus. New York, NY, USA: Raven Press; 1993. pp. 107-172

[115] McKenzie J, El-Guindy A. Epstein-Barr virus lytic cycle reactivation. Current Topics in Microbiology and Immunology. 2015;**391**:237-261. DOI: 10.1007/978-3-319-22834-1_8

[116] Tsao SW, Tsang CM, Lo KW. Epstein-Barr virus infection and nasopharyngeal carcinoma. Philosophical Transactions of the Royal Society of London. Series B, Biological Sciences. 2017;**372**(1732):20160270. DOI: 10.1098/rstb.2016.0270

[117] Guidry JT, Birdwell CE, Scott RS. Epstein-Barr virus in the pathogenesis of oral cancers. Oral Diseases. 2018;**24**(4):497-508. DOI: 10.1111/odi.12656. Epub 2017 Apr 18

[118] Andersson J. An overview of Epstein-Barr virus: From discovery to future directions for treatment and prevention herpes. 2000;**7**(3):76-82. Available from: https://pubmed.ncbi.nlm.nih.gov/11867007/

[119] Epstein MA, Achong BG. Introduction: Discovery and general biology of the virus. In: Epstein MA, Achong BG, editors. The Epstein-Barr virus. Berlin Heidelberg New York: Springer; 1979. pp. 1-22

[120] Sixbey JW, Shirley P, Chesney PJ, Buntin DM, Resnick L. Detection of a second widespread strain of Epstein-Barr virus. Lancet. 1989;**2**(8666):761-765. DOI: 10.1016/s0140-6736(89)90829-5

[121] Bricháček B, Hirsch I, Síbl O, Vilikusová E, Vonka V. Association of some supraglottic laryngeal carcinomas with EB virus. International Journal of Cancer. 1983;**32**(2):193-197. DOI: 10.1002/ijc.2910320209

[122] de Lima MAP, Silva ÁDL, do Nascimento Filho ACS, Cordeiro TL, JPS B, MAB R, et al. Epstein-Barr virus-associated carcinoma of the larynx: A systematic review with meta-analysis. Pathogens. 2021;**10**(11):1429. DOI: 10.3390/pathogens10111429

[123] Cathomas G. Kaposi's sarcoma-associated herpesvirus (KSHV)/ human herpesvirus 8 (HHV-8) as a tumour virus. Herpes. 2003;**10**(3):72-77. Available from: https://pubmed.ncbi.nlm.nih.gov/14759339/

[124] Stanberry LR. Herpes Viruses. In: International Encyclopedia of Public Health. Amsterdam, The Netherlands: Elsevier; 2008. pp. 382-389

[125] Dittmer DP, Damania B. Kaposi sarcoma associated herpesvirus pathogenesis (KSHV)–an update.

Current Opinion in Virology. 2013;**3**(3):238-244. DOI: 10.1016/j.coviro.2013.05.012. Epub 2013 Jun 13

[126] Bhatt AP, Damania B. AKTivation of PI3K/AKT/mTOR signaling pathway by KSHV. Frontiers in Immunology. 2013;**3**:401. DOI: 10.3389/fimmu.2012.00401

[127] Nador RG, Cesarman E, Chadburn A, Dawson DB, Ansari MQ, Sald J, et al. Primary effusion lymphoma: A distinct clinicopathologic entity associated with the Kaposi's sarcoma-associated herpes virus. Blood. 1996;**88**(2):645-656. Available from: https://pubmed.ncbi.nlm.nih.gov/8695812/

[128] Huang G, Low G. Human herpes Virus-8-associated multicentric Castleman's disease in a human immunodeficiency virus-positive patient with a previous history of Kaposi's sarcoma. Journal of Clinical Imaging Science. 2015;**5**:59. DOI: 10.4103/2156-7514.168713

[129] Güvenç MG, Midilli K, Ozdoğan A, Inci E, Tahamiler R, Enver O, et al. Detection of HHV-8 and HPV in laryngeal carcinoma. Auris, Nasus, Larynx. 2008;**35**(3):357-362. DOI: 10.1016/j.anl.2007.08.006. Epub 2007 Oct 30

[130] Parker TM, Smith EM, Ritchie JM, Haugen TH, Vonka V, Turek LP, et al. Head and neck cancer associated with herpes simplex virus 1 and 2 and other risk factors. Oral Oncology. 2006;**42**(3):288-296. DOI: 10.1016/j.oraloncology.2005.08.003

[131] Koivikko T, Rodrigues PC, Vehviläinen M, Hyvönen P, Sundquist E, Arffman RK, et al. Detection of herpes simplex virus in oral tongue squamous cell carcinoma. Frontiers in Pharmacology. 2023;**14**:1182152. DOI: 10.3389/fphar.2023.1182152

[132] von Stebut J, Heiland M, Preissner R, Rendenbach C, Preissner S. Association of Herpes simplex infection with significantly increased risk of head and neck cancer: Real-world evidence of about 500,000 patients. International Journal of Dermatology. 2024. DOI: 10.1111/ijd.17196. Epub ahead of print

[133] Trivic A, Milovanovic J, Kablar D, Tomic A, Folic M, Jotic A, et al. Friend or foe? Exploring the role of cytomegalovirus (HCMV) infection in head and neck Tumors. Biomedicine. 2024;**12**(4):872. DOI: 10.3390/biomedicines12040872

[134] Wołącewicz M, Becht R, Grywalska E, Niedźwiedzka-Rystwej P. Herpesviruses in head and neck cancers. Viruses. 2020;**12**(2):172. DOI: 10.3390/v12020172

[135] Kim M, Lee YK, Park B, Oh DJ, Choi HG. Hepatitis virus B and C infections are associated with an increased risk of non-Hodgkin lymphoma: A nested case-control study using a national sample cohort. Journal of Medical Virology. 2020;**92**(8):1214-1220. DOI: 10.1002/jmv.25653. Epub 2019 Dec 19

[136] Gondivkar SM, Parikh RV, Gadbail AR, Solanke V, Chole R, Mankar M, et al. Involvement of viral factors with head and neck cancers. Oral Oncology. 2012;**48**(3):195-199. DOI: 10.1016/j.oraloncology.2011.10.007. Epub 2011 Nov 9

[137] Hettmann A, Demcsák A, Decsi G, Bach Á, Pálinkó D, Rovó L, et al. Infectious agents associated with head and neck carcinomas. Advances in Experimental Medicine

and Biology. 2016;**897**:63-80. DOI: 10.1007/5584_2015_5005

[138] Tsai KN, Kuo CF, Ou JJ. Mechanisms of hepatitis B virus persistence. Trends in Microbiology. 2018;**26**(1):33-42. DOI: 10.1016/j.tim.2017.07.006. Epub 2017 Aug 16

[139] McGivern DR, Lemon SM. Virus-specific mechanisms of carcinogenesis in hepatitis C virus associated liver cancer. Oncogene. 2011;**30**(17):1969-1983. DOI: 10.1038/onc.2010.594. Epub 2011 Jan 24

[140] Guntaka Ramareddy V, Padala Mythili K. Interaction of hepatitis C viral proteins with cellular oncoproteins in the induction of liver cancer. International Scholarly Research Notices. 2014:351407

[141] Donà S, Borsetto D, Fussey J, Biscaro V, Vian E, Spinato G, et al. Association between hepatitis C and B viruses and head and neck squamous cell carcinoma. Journal of Clinical Virology. 2019;**121**:104209. DOI: 10.1016/j.jcv.2019.104209. Epub 2019 Nov 4

[142] Nayyar SS, Thiagarajan S, Malik A, D'Cruz A, Chaukar D, Patil P, et al. Head and neck squamous cell carcinoma in HIV, HBV and HCV seropositive patients - prognosis and its predictors. Journal of Cancer Research and Therapeutics. 2020;**16**(3):619-623. DOI: 10.4103/jcrt.JCRT_166_19

[143] Komori MF, Kimura T, Kariya S, Onoda T, Takeda S, Mizukawa N, et al. Epidemiological correlations between head and neck cancer and hepatitis B core antibody positivity. Anticancer Research. 2020;**40**(4):2393-2403. DOI: 10.21873/anticanres.14209

[144] Su TH, Tseng TC, Liu CJ, Chou SW, Liu CH, Yang HC, et al. Antiviral therapy against chronic hepatitis C is associated with a reduced risk of oral cancer. International Journal of Cancer. 2020;**147**(3):901-908. DOI: 10.1002/ijc.32840. Epub 2020 Jan 2

[145] Borsetto D, Fussey J, Fabris L, Bandolin L, Gaudioso P, Phillips V, et al. HCV infection and the risk of head and neck cancer: A meta-analysis. Oral Oncology. 2020;**109**:104869. DOI: 10.1016/j.oraloncology.2020.104869. Epub ahead of print

[146] Hung SH, Yang TH, Cheng YF, Chen CS, Lin HC. Associations of head and neck cancer with hepatitis B virus and hepatitis C virus infection. Cancers (Basel). 2023;**15**(18):4510. DOI: 10.3390/cancers15184510

[147] Tan R, Zhu X, Sun Y, Yang S, Peng C, Feng X, et al. The association of HBV infection and head and neck cancer: A systematic review and meta-analysis. BMC Cancer. 2024;**24**(1):225. DOI: 10.1186/s12885-024-11967-7

[148] Lai CL, Lin CH, Su YC, Shih YH, Wang CC, Teng CJ, et al. Survival outcomes of patients with head and neck squamous cell cancer with hepatitis B virus infection: An analysis from an endemic tertiary center. Cancer Medicine. 2023;**12**(6):6802-6810. DOI: 10.1002/cam4.5469. Epub 2022 Nov 24

[149] Poluschkin L, Rautava J, Turunen A, Wang Y, Hedman K, Syrjänen K, et al. Polyomaviruses detectable in head and neck carcinomas. Oncotarget. 2018;**9**(32):22642-22652. DOI: 10.18632/oncotarget.25202

[150] Mohebbi E, Noormohamadi Z, Sadeghi-Rad H, Sadeghi F, Yahyapour Y, Vaziri F, et al. Low viral load of Merkel cell polyomavirus in Iranian patients with head and neck squamous cell carcinoma: Is it clinically important? Journal of

Medical Virology. 2018;**90**(2):344-350. DOI: 10.1002/jmv.24953. Epub 2017 Oct 20

[151] Muñoz JP, Blanco R, Osorio JC, Oliva C, Diaz MJ, Carrillo-Beltrán D, et al. Merkel cell polyomavirus detected in head and neck carcinomas from Chile. Infectious Agents and Cancer. 2020;**15**:4. DOI: 10.1186/s13027-020-0276-z

[152] Hasani Estalkhi M, Seyed Majidi M, Sadeghi F, Chehrazi M, Zebardast A, Hasanzadeh A, et al. Prevalence of Merkel cell polyomavirus (MCPyV) in the oral cavity biopsies in northern Iran. Asian Pacific Journal of Cancer Prevention. 2021;**22**(12):3927-3932. DOI: 10.31557/APJCP.2021.22.12.3927

[153] Beachler DC, D'Souza G. Oral human papillomavirus infection and head and neck cancers in HIV-infected individuals. Current Opinion in Oncology. 2013;**25**(5):503-510. DOI: 10.1097/CCO.0b013e32836242b4

[154] Salahuddin S, Cohen O, Wu M, Irizarry JP, Vega T, Gan G, et al. Impact of HIV infection on clinical outcomes among people diagnosed with head and neck cancer. Journal of Clinical Oncology. 2022;**40**:e18080

[155] Yusuf K, Sampath V, Umar S. Bacterial infections and cancer: Exploring this association and its implications for cancer patients. International Journal of Molecular Sciences. 2023;**24**(4):3110. DOI: 10.3390/ijms24043110

[156] Wroblewski LE, Peek RM Jr, Wilson KT. *Helicobacter pylori* and gastric cancer: Factors that modulate disease risk. Clinical Microbiology Reviews. 2010;**23**(4):713-739. DOI: 10.1128/CMR.00011-10

[157] Irani S, Barati I, Badiei M. Periodontitis and oral cancer - current concepts of the etiopathogenesis. Oncology Reviews. 2020;**14**(1):465. DOI: 10.4081/oncol.2020.465

[158] Chattopadhyay I, Verma M, Panda M. Role of oral microbiome signatures in diagnosis and prognosis of oral cancer. Technology in Cancer Research & Treatment. 2019;**18**:1533033819867354. DOI: 10.1177/1533033819867354

[159] Baima G, Minoli M, Michaud DS, Aimetti M, Sanz M, Loos BG, et al. Periodontitis and risk of cancer: Mechanistic evidence. Periodontology 2000. 2000;**2023**. DOI: 10.1111/prd.12540. Epub ahead of print

[160] Polz-Gruszka D, Stec A, Dworzański J, Polz-Dacewicz M. EBV, HSV, CMV and HPV in laryngeal and oropharyngeal carcinoma in polish patients. Anticancer Research. 2015;**35**(3):1657-1661. Available from: https://ar.iiarjournals.org/content/35/3/1657.long

[161] Vanshika S, Preeti A, Sumaira Q, Vijay K, Shikha T, Shivanjali R, et al. Incidence of HPV and EBV in oral cancer and their clinico-pathological correlation- a pilot study of 108 cases. Journal of Oral Biology and Craniofacial Research. 2021;**11**(2):180-184. DOI: 10.1016/j.jobcr.2021.01.007. Epub 2021 Jan 23

[162] Blanco R, Carrillo-Beltrán D, Corvalán AH, Aguayo F. High-risk human papillomavirus and Epstein-Barr virus coinfection: A potential role in head and neck carcinogenesis. Biology (Basel). 2021;**10**(12):1232. DOI: 10.3390/biology10121232

[163] Migliaro M, Massuh D, Infante MF, Brahm AM, San Martín MT, Ortuño D. Role of Epstein-Barr virus and human papilloma virus in the development

of oropharyngeal cancer: A literature review. International Journal of Dentistry. 2022;**2022**:3191569. DOI: 10.1155/2022/3191569

[164] Al-Thawadi H, Gupta I, Jabeen A, Skenderi F, Aboulkassim T, Yasmeen A, et al. Co-presence of human papillomaviruses and Epstein-Barr virus is linked with advanced tumor stage: A tissue microarray study in head and neck cancer patients. Cancer Cell International. 2020;**20**:361. DOI: 10.1186/s12935-020-01348-y

[165] Ursu RG, Luchian I, Ghetu N, Costan VV, Stamatin O, Palade OD, et al. Emerging oncogenic viruses in head and neck cancers from Romanian patients. Applied Sciences. 2021;**11**(19):9356. DOI: 10.3390/app11199356

[166] Mulder FJ, Klufah F, Janssen FME, Farshadpour F, Willems SM, de Bree R, et al. Presence of human papillomavirus and Epstein-Barr virus, but absence of Merkel cell polyomavirus, in head and neck cancer of non-smokers and non-drinkers. Frontiers in Oncology. 2021;**10**:560434. DOI: 10.3389/fonc.2020.560434

[167] Schindele A, Holm A, Nylander K, Allard A, Olofsson K. Mapping human papillomavirus, Epstein-Barr virus, cytomegalovirus, adenovirus, and p16 in laryngeal cancer. Discover Oncology. 2022;**13**(1):18. DOI: 10.1007/s12672-022-00475-4

[168] Yu C, Li L, Wang S, Xu Y, Wang L, Huang Y, et al. Advances in nanomaterials for the diagnosis and treatment of head and neck cancers: A review. Bioactive Materials. 2023;**25**:430-444. ISSN 2452-199X. DOI: 10.1016/j.bioactmat.2022.08.010

Chapter 6

Recent Treatment Trends of Chronic Rhinosinusitis (CRS): According to Phenotype and Endotype

Joon Kon Kim

Abstract

Chronic rhinosinusitis is a major ENT disease that makes daily life uncomfortable. Symptoms of chronic rhinosinusitis often include nasal congestion, purulent rhinorrhea, postnasal drip, and olfactory impairment. If symptoms persist, medical treatment, which is a reversible method, or surgical treatment, which is an irreversible method that structurally changes the paranasal cavity, could be considered. Currently, antibiotics with mucociliary agents can be used as typical medical treatment, and sinus irrigation with saline solution may also be considered. Surgical treatment is commonly performed through endoscopic sinus surgery, and an open approach can also be considered for structures that are difficult to access. For refractory CRS that does not respond to phenotype-specific treatment, the treatment is performed by examining the endotypes of CRS. Treatment based on the representative endotype checks the presence or absence of type 2 inflammation and provides customized treatment using biologics and hormonal treatment accordingly.

Keywords: chronic rhinosinusitis, recent treatment, medical treatment, surgical treatment, phenotype, endotype

1. Introduction

It is important to understand immune cells and cytokines-related pathway for clarifying chronic rhinosinusitis (CRS) occurrence mechanism. Diverse immune cells such as T cells, antigen-presenting cells, and innate lymphocyte cells are involved in the CRS generation. Progressing CRS serially, sinonasal mucosa remodeling is developed and nasal polyp is often formed by a synchronization of sinonasal immunity and cross-linked fibrin deposition.

2. Chronic rhinosinusitis

CRS is defined by an inflammation of the paranasal mucosa with olfactory symptoms such as anosmia and hyposmia, nasal obstruction, rhinorrhea, and facial pain lasting more than 12 weeks. In general, CRS occurs in 5–12% of the global population [1].

Phenotype of CRS is classified into CRS without nasal polyps (CRSsNP) and CRS with nasal polyps (CRSwNP). CRSwNP can be divided into eosinophilic CRSwNP (eosCRSwNP) or non-eosinophilic CRSwNP (non-eosCRSwNP) according to the eosinophil levels of the polyp tissues.

CRS is diagnosed by medical history, physical examination with nasal endoscopy, and mucosal inflammation of radiological evaluation. There are diverse methods of treatments of CRS such as topical nasal sprays, nasal irrigation, antibiotics, steroids, immunomodulators, and surgical treatments. According to the guideline of worldwide consensus, for example, European Position Paper on Chronic Rhinosinusitis and Nasal Polyps 2020 (EPOS2020) and European Forum for Research and Education in Allergy and Airway Diseases (EUFOREA), the treatment of CRS can be done step by step. In case of failure of CRS treatment, biologics were used successfully as additional treatment option for an improvement in the quality of life.

3. CRS pathophysiology

The mechanisms related to CRS pathogenesis connect to each other between immunity and environmental factors. Exogenous factors that are pathogens such as bacteria, viruses, and fungi as well as external environmental materials such as allergens and air pollutants trigger a commencement of the protection of nasal cavity/paranasal sinus at the cell-immune level. This protective immune mechanism occurs with innate immunity and adaptive immunity serially. The immunities are involved in epithelial proinflammatory cytokine production, toll-like receptors (TLRs) activation, chemo-sensory cell activation, and mucociliary clearance. After repeated immunologic defense, the nasal cavity and paranasal sinus change to chronic inflammation state. There is cell tight junction disruption, tissue remodeling, and bacteria dysbiosis in a chronic inflammation. The immunological changes manifest into forms such as nasal obstruction, rhinorrhea, and loss of smell.

To categorize CRS endotyping, T lymphocyte is classified according to several types of T lymphocyte and T lymphocyte–producing cytokines. T lymphocyte is classified into T1, T2, and T3. T1 type produces IFN-γ representatively, and T1 type has additional cytokines that are CXCL9, CXCL11, GZMG, ZNF683, FCRL6, and SLCO1B3. IFN-γ is presented by Th1 cells, cytotoxic T cells, and group 1 innate lymphocyte cells (ILC1s). T2 type secretes IL-4, IL-5, IL-13, EPX, CCL18, CCL26, CCR3, CST1, CST2, CLCA1, FCER2, POSTIN, PTGDR2, and SIGLEC8. These cytokines are also shown by Th2 cells, ILC2s, and eosinophils. T3 type is characterized by IL-17A. IL-17A is shown by Th17 cells and ILC3s. T3 type possesses other cytokines that are IL1B, IL8, CXCL1, CXCL2, CXCL6, CCL20, CHI3L1, SAA1, SAA2, and NOX1 [2]. According to the published literatures, these endotypes can match each patient, and some patients may have mixed endotypes (T1-T2, T2-T3, and T1-T3). There are few people who do not express elevated levels of any kind of biomarkers [3]. Patients having this characteristic are T untypeable (Tun). T2 type is usually presented in patients with CRSwNP, and non-T2 type (T1 or T3) is seen in patients with CRSwNP. Western countries have T2 type-CRSwNP more than Asian countries. Because of different immunological and environmental factors from Western/Asian countries, there is disparate bacterial entity in the CRS. To differentiate CRS types, CRS can be divided into eosinophilic, neutrophilic, pauci-granulocytic, and granulocytic.

Phenotypic classification is determined from the presence or absence of nasal polyps, and comorbidities define the phenotypic classification [4]. Nasal cavity and paranasal sinus mucosa have an important function to differentiate CRS, and epithelial cells of mucosa play a crucial role that is associated with the initiation and regulation of immune responses. CD4+ T cell expansion corresponds to raising up type 2 cytokines and immunoglobulins in NPs [5].

4. Phenotypes of CRS

CRS is chronic inflammation of the mucosa from the nasal cavity/paranasal sinuses. CRS affects up to 12% of the Western population [6]. According to EPOS 2020 guidelines, CRS is diagnosed by the confirmation of 2 or more symptoms for 12 weeks or more continuous weeks with objective confirmation using computed tomography (CT) and nasal endoscopy. CRS phenotypes are divided according to nasal polyp existence and nonexistence because of different CRS treatment courses: CRS with nasal polyps (CRSwNP) and CRS without nasal polyps (CRSsNP). In addition to CRSwNP and CRSsNP, there were other observable characteristics of CRS phenotypes.

4.1 Aspirin-exacerbated respiratory disease (AERD)

AERD is defined by three characteristics that are (1) nasal polyp, (2) asthma, and (3) sensitivity to cyclooxygenase type 1 inhibitors. Respiratory airway symptoms are aggravated by blocking cyclooxygenase type 1. Aspirin and other nonsteroidal anti-inflammatory drugs (NSAIDs) bring about this blocking reaction. Actually, AERD generation does not reveal entirely. There is high production of cysteinyl leukotrienes and prostaglandin D2 with lower levels of prostaglandin E2 with increased eosinophil activation. The prevalence of AERD among adult asthma patients has been reported to range between 7 and 21%, whereas 9–16% of patients with CRSwNP have been identified as having AERD [7, 8]. AERD is usually presented to be more prevalent in the Western countries than in Asian countries. The clinical diagnosis of AERD is confirmed by the presence of nasal polyps, asthma, and sensitivity to cyclooxygenase type 1 inhibitors. AERD occurs at a younger age and with a more severe clinical presentation compared with the typical patient with nasal polyposis [9]. AERD is confirmed by a history taking from a patient who experienced aspirin and NSAID hypersensitivity. Because aspirin and NSAID hypersensitivity can be gradual, it may not be easily recognized. Symptoms of AERD such as rhinorrhea, nasal obstruction, epiphora, conjunctival edema, laryngospasm, or bronchospasm typically occur within hours after the administration of aspirin and NSAIDs. Stevens WW et al. and Mascia K et al. showed that AERD patients have significantly decreased FEV1 relative to other CRS patients with asthma [7, 10]. Treatment of AERD can include aggressive surgery. Other treatments such as newly available biologics and ASA desensitization can be applied as alternatives.

4.2 Allergic fungal rhinosinusitis

Allergic fungal rhinosinusitis (AFRS) is an IgE-mediated noninvasive fungal disease of the nasal and paranasal sinuses. It occurs in less than 10% of CRSwNP cases. Patients with AFRS are also more likely to have lower socioeconomic status based on the results from retrospective studies [11]. The general symptoms of AFRS are rhinorrhea, nasal obstruction, and decreased sense of smell, and the severe symptoms of the disease are visual changes, proptosis, headaches, and diplopia. The symptoms usually present unilaterally. During the endoscopic evaluation of AFRS, there are thick brownish allergic mucins that have a peanut butter–like appearance with nasal polyps and proteinaceous debris. There are eosinophils and fungal hyphae, evaluating the content of AFRS mucin. Bent and Kuhn [12] represents the criteria to confirm AFRS. The major criteria of AFRS are (1) nasal polyposis, (2) fungi on staining, (3) eosinophilic mucin without fungal invasion into sinus tissue, (4) type 1 hypersensitivity of fungi, and (5) characteristic radiological findings with soft tissue differential densities on CT scanning. And, The minor criteria of AFRS are (1) bone erosion, (2) Charcot-Leyden crystals, (3) unilateral disease, (4) type 1 hypersensitivity to fungi, and (5) positive fungal culture. The appropriate treatment of AFRS is surgical approach with corticosteroid treatment.

4.3 Eosinophilic granulomatosis with polyangiitis

Eosinophilic granulomatosis with polyangiitis (EGPA, so-called Churg-Strauss syndrome) is a rare disease, which is involved in the small-vessel vasculitis-affected asthma and eosinophilia. The incidence of EGPA is 0.5–6.8 cases per 1,000,000 adults per year occurring most often in adults aged 40–60 years of age [13]. The progress of EGPA has three phases: allergic, eosinophilic, and vasculitic. Allergic phase presents with symptoms of asthma, allergic rhinitis, and sinusitis. And, eosinophilic phase shows blood and tissue eosinophilia. Vasculitic phase displays the abnormal vascular disorder such as peripheral neuropathy, purpura, and pauci-immune necrotizing glomerulonephritis. EGPA usually has the comorbidity of asthma. The representative symptoms of EGPA are nasal obstruction, rhinorrhea, smell dysfunction, and sneezing. In the published papers, there is no appropriate diagnosis of EGPA. As an alternative diagnosis, pathological biopsy identified vasculitis/eosinophilic inflammatory process even if the biopsy is not useful to make a diagnosis. According to the symptoms of EGPA, conservative treatment can be done such as nasal saline irrigation or topical intranasal steroid treatment. Surgical treatment is not recommended, and biological medication (i.e., IL-5 receptor-targeting agent) can be chosen.

4.4 Cystic fibrosis

Cystic fibrosis (CF) is a benign disease, which inherits autosomal-recessive characteristics. CF is a defect, which is derived from the cystic fibrosis transmembrane receptor (CFTR) gene through chloride channels. CF expresses significantly the increase of nasal secretion in the upper and lower airways prohibiting mucociliary function. Therefore, there is a high risk of infections. On radiologic imaging, CF patients have a higher incidence of underdeveloped sinuses compared with other adult patients. CF is diagnosed by performing a sweat chloride test, genetic analysis, and clinical presentation. A sweat chloride test is done by spotting a solution on the forearm or thigh and doing electrical stimulation, which is related to sweating. While examining the chloride, the level of chloride of CF should be higher than that in a normal patient. And, CF is verified by evaluating the CFTR mutation for the genetic test.

4.5 Immunodeficiency

Patients with refractory CRS continuously should be considered for immunodeficiency. Immunodeficient patients with CRS can be further categorized as having a primary or secondary immunodeficiency. Primary immunodeficiency is direct defect of immune response such as B cell, T cell, and other immune cell dysfunction. Secondary immunodeficiency is a result of indirect influence related to other diseases such as HIV or chemotherapy. The CRS-influenced immunodeficiency can be difficult to mark off idiopathic CRS. Therefore, meticulous history taking and evaluation should be chosen. Characteristic of immunodeficiency-related CRS is the rapid recurrence of symptoms and nasal polyps. The representative immunodeficiency is IgA immunodeficiency. There are other immunodeficiencies such as IgG and IgM immunodeficiency.

4.6 Primary ciliary dyskinesia

Normal mucosa of nasal cavity and paranasal sinus is pseudostratified columnar-ciliated epithelium. Primary ciliary dyskinesia (PCD) impairs the cilia movement. Symptoms of PCD are nasal obstruction and rhinorrhea because of static mucociliary function. PCD is a rare disorder with the incidence estimated at 1:15,000–30,000 births [14]. Saccharin test is the method to evaluate PCD. Saccharin test checks the nasal flow time from inferior turbinate to nasopharynx compared with normal nasal mucosa flow. In the case of delayed nasal flow of saccharin test, PCD can be diagnosed. There is also another screening test for PCD, nasal nitric oxide test that checks lower levels of nitric oxide of nasal cavity and paranasal sinus.

5. Reboot surgery

CRS accompanied by asthma, AERD, and atopy has a higher recurrence rate of CRS.

Refractory CRSwNP is treated by recurrent surgical treatments to deal with the recurrence of pathologic lesions. The concept of surgical approach changes from simple polyp extraction to the recovery of sinonasal mucosal function. Because of the high recurrence rates of CRSwNP, more extended approaches are proposed for new concepts such as (1) to widely access the sinuses, (2) to open them for local treatment, and (3) to reduce the inflammatory load. Actually, "stripping of the mucosa" procedure is not recommended because of the fear of scarring, inflammation of the denuded bone, and non-functional mucosa [15]. But CRSwNP is characterized by the high recurrence of disease morbidity and more systemic disease tendency than CRSwNP. Sinus surgery for CRSwNP should be performed to improve the quality of life and the patient's symptoms. So, "reboot surgery" is introduced to advance CRSwNP treatment effect, recently. The main point of reboot surgery is to remove the sinus mucosa inflammation entirely. After this surgical approach, there is the recovery of sinonasal mucosa grown from preserved normal mucosa within several weeks. The range of the procedure is to remove totally the ethmoid sinus and maxillary sinus mucosa adding the orbital lamina and skull base mucosa. Furthermore, in the case of CRSwNP extended to the frontal sinus, a Draft 3 procedure should be considered. "Full reboot surgery" is the procedure of removing the maxillary sinus, ethmoid sinus, and frontal sinus mucosa, otherwise, "partial reboot."

The reboot technique begins with a middle meatal antrostomy widely and a complete removal of all the mucosa from the maxillary sinus including the alveolar recess mucosa. In the case of the pathologic lesion extended to lamina orbitalis, skull base, and the lateral aspects of the middle turbinate, the mucosa of these structures is stripped. Additionally, sphenoid sinus lesion is needed for very careful reboot surgery owing to critical structures such as internal carotid artery and optic nerve. The range of reboot surgery at the sphenoid sinus is the floor and medial parts of the sphenoid sinus.

For an example of frontal sinus, the procedure is done by removing the anterior skull base mucosa and is performed by widening the frontal sinus opening. Middle turbinate should be preserved as a landmark of postoperative care. Superior turbinate should also be protected, but in the case of blocking the surgical route, this structure can be removed. And, Draf III procedure is performed to achieve a full reboot surgery. The frontal sinus mucosa is completely removed from the posterior and anterior walls. "Peering of the sinus mucosa" derives from the concept that there is a nasal mucosa growth over the sinus walls from the edges of the anterior nasal cavity and the inferior turbinate, and there is no remnant paranasal mucosa. Mucosa recovery is 4–6 weeks, but there is a delay of epithelization of mucosa in a situation with infection. For example, type 2 inflammation causes the delay of mucosa healing because type 2 inflammation-producing cytokines such as IL-4 and IL-13 weaken epithelial tight junction expression [16].

Complication rate of reboot surgery is identical to the rate of endoscopic sinus surgery (ESS). In the case adjacent to lamina orbitalis/skull base, fine surgical movement should be chosen to avoid a complication. Checking the SNOT-22 after reboot surgery is a useful method for an evaluation of surgical result. Recovery time of smell postoperatively usually is several weeks unless there is critical olfactory nerve complication.

6. Surgery outcome and predictors

ESS is an appropriate treatment to solve CRSwNP and CRSsNP. But ESS is not a perfect resolution to these diseases because of some recurrence rates. To predict a result of ESS success, there are diverse parameters of prediction, for example, postoperative smell outcome, quality of life improvement, and postoperative polyp recurrence/sinusitis rate. According to these predictive parameters, long-term postoperative follow-up can be evaluated and improve quality of life postoperatively.

6.1 Symptoms and quality-of-life improvement and prediction

In published literatures, there are improvements in quality of life (QOL) and nasal symptoms following ESS. Most of these studies are non-randomized uncontrolled (level III), and only few randomized controlled trials are available [17].

6.2 Polyp recurrence and revision surgery and prediction

To predict a polyp recurrence, it is useful to check a mucosal eosinophilia. There is no appropriate consensus of eosinophilic CRS tissue eosinophilia definition. To define tissue eosinophilia, there are diverse criteria in literature. Some papers present that eosinophilic CRS is related to eosinophil count/HPF (400xmagnification). The eosinophil count/HPF of papers defines various measurement as a cutoff value of eosinophilic sinusitis. For example, there are "5" [18], "20" [19], "70" [20], "100" [21], and "120" [22] that are cutoff values of eosinophilic sinusitis. Another evaluation of eosinophilic sinusitis is to check the proportion of eosinophil cells. In general, most studying groups evaluate 10% as the proportion-cutoff value. The other evaluation of eosinophilic sinusitis is to assess the clinical data such as serum eosinophil count (>5%), ethmoid predominant lesion by CT, comorbidity of asthma, and NSAID intolerance. Additionally, there are other clinical parameters such as the ratio of total ethmoid sinus scores and maxillary sinus scores for both sides (E/M ratio) and polypoid changes of the middle turbinate to predict polyp recurrence [23]. There are also other prediction parameters, for example, Charcot-Leyden crystal (CLC), eosinophil cationic protein (ECP), eotaxin-3, periostin, and IL-5.

7. Biologics in chronic rhinosinusitis with nasal polyps

In cases of recalcitrant CRSwNP, postoperative recurrent CRSwNP, and uncontrolled severe CRSNP, there is poor efficacy of diverse treatment despite medical and surgical approaches (topical nasal glucocorticosteroid, oral glucocorticosteroid, and endoscopic sinus surgery). Additionally, there are fewer effective outcomes in a case with asthma. Gevaert P et al. showed omalizumab, a new treatment agent for severe asthma, targets free IgE. This agent prevents binding to IgE receptors. The coverage of omalizumab expanded to CRSwNP [24]. Proof-of-concept studies with reslizumab and mepolizumab (biologics against IL-5) in CRSwNP were done in 2006/2011. This study's results actually focused on asthma than on CRSwNP. Benralizumab also targets IL-5 and functions an anti-IL-5 receptor antagonist. Dupilumab is an anti-IL-4 receptor antagonist, the first biologic for the indication of CRSwNP. Phase 2 and 3 studies are related to dupilumab published [9, 25] (**Table 1**). Biologics, for example, mepolizumab, omalizumab, and dupilumab, can considerably reduce the nasal polyp score, Lund-Mackay CT score, and nasal and sinus symptoms. Evaluating SNOT-22, there is an improvement of score following the use of biologics (**Table 2**). In cases of CRSwNP with comorbidity such as asthma, biologics such as dupilumab and omalizumab can increase lung function and asthma control. The mechanism of biologics is to reduce blood/tissue eosinophils and serum IgE levels. For example, dupilumab reduces type 2 inflammation in polyp tissue and the polyp size in polyp tissue. Dupilumab presented that antagonism of IL-4Rα signaling suppresses type 2 cytokine-dependent process, such as mucosal IgE formation, the expression of chemokines attracting inflammatory cells [27].

7.1 IL-5 targeting agent

Biologics associated with IL-5 are reslizumab and mepolizumab. IL-5 is released by innate lymphoid cells (ILC2), Th2 cells, mast cells, γδ-T cells, and eosinophils. IL-5 binds to the α subunit of the IL-5 receptor (IL-5Rα) in the transmembrane form and soluble form. Reslizumab and mepolizumab act to retain IL-5 in serum and mucosal tissues. The action is important for the migration, chemotaxis and recruitment, activation, proliferation, maturation, and survival of eosinophil [28]. For example, benralizumab is an anti-IL-5 treatment agent that is a humanized mAb that binds with high affinity to the α-chain of the human IL-5R. The function of this agent is to block IL 5R activation and signal transduction. Benralizumab attaches to FcgR receptor that elevates the antibody-dependent cell-mediated cytotoxicity (ADCC) function [29].

7.2 IgE targeting agent

The biologic associated with IgE is omalizumab, representatively. Immunoglobulin E (IgE) antibodies are mediated by allergic reaction and function through binding to Fc receptors FcεRI on mast cells basophils, and dendritic

	Mepolizumab	Omalizumab	Dupilumab	Mepolizumab
Year	2011	2013	2016, 2019	2017
Target molecule	IL-5	IgE	IL-4 receptor alpha	IL-5
Study design[a]	Single center	Two centers	Multicenter (13 sites)	Multicenter (6 sites)
NO. (verum/ placebo)	30 (20/10)	23 (15/8)	60 (30/30)	105 (54/51)
Asthma % (verum/ placebo)	43% (50%/30%)	100% (100%/100%)	58% (63%/53%)	78% (81%/75%)
Former surgery % (verum/ placebo)	77% (75%/80%)	83% (87%/75%)	58% (63%/ 53%)	100% (100%/100%)
End point and last visit (weeks)	8w/48w	16w/20w	16w/16w	25w/25w
Therapeutic effects	Significant reduction of polyp scores; reduction of blood eosinophil counts, serum ECP, and IL-5Rα, IL-6, MPO in nasal secretion	Significant reduction of polyp and CT scores, and improvement of symptoms of upper and lower airway and AQLQ	Significant reduction of polyp and CT scores, and improvement of smelling, symptoms, and quality of life (SNOT-22); improvement of FEV1 and ACQ5. Reduced plasma eotaxin-3, serum and nasal secretion tIgE, and nasal tissue tIgE, IL13, ECP, PARK, Eotaxin 1,2,3	Significant reduction of polyp score, and improvement of smelling, symptoms, and quality of life (SNOT-22)

[a]All these studies were randomized, double-blind, placebo-controlled studies.
tIgE: total serum immunoglobulin E; AQLQ: Asthma Quality of Life Questionnaire; ACQ5: 5-item Asthma Control Questionnaire, PnIF: Peak Nasal Inspiratory Flow, FEV1: forced expiratory volume; SNOT-22: Sino-nasal outcome test-22; ECP: eosinophil cationic protein; IL-5Rα: IL-5: receptor α subunit; TARC: Thymus and Activation-Regulated Chemokine; PARK: pulmonary and activation-regulated chemokine; MPO: myeloperoxidase. Table 1. refers to Zhang and Bachert [9].

Table 1.
Biologics information developed in the recent real-world field.

cells and FcεRII/CD23 on B cells. After IgE stimulation, antigen-presenting cells (APCs) act in serial response with leukotrienes, prostaglandins, IL-4, IL-5, and IL-13. This continual cascade mechanism results in eosinophil aggregation. Omalizumab antagonizes IgE-related reaction of APCs. IgE functions to induce mast cell mediators that maintain the inflammatory reaction [30]. Gevaert P et al. show that omalizumab has a positive effect to treat respiratory tract infection regardless of allergy [24]. This study was designed by a randomized, double-blind, placebo-controlled trial of allergic and non-allergic patients with nasal polyps and comorbid asthma. In the study, there were two groups that are omalizumab treatment group and placebo group (omalizumab, n = 16; placebo, n = 8). Nasal polyp score of endoscopic exam and Lund-Mackay score of CT were used in the study.

Characteristic pattern	Dupilumab	Mepolizumab	Omalizumab
CRSwNP			
Reduction of endoscopic nasal polyp score	O	O	O
Lund-Mackay CT scan score improvement	O	-	O
Reduction of relevant nasal symptoms	O	O	O
Increase in smell (UPSIT and VAS)	O	O	O
Increase in quality of life (SNOT-22)	O	O	O
Asthma			
Increase in lung function (FEV1)	O	-	O
Asthma control (ACQ and AQLQ)	O	-	O
Biomarker			
Reduction in blood eosinophil numbers	-	O	-
Reduction in serum IgE levels	O	-	O
Reduction in tissue eosinophil numbers	O	O	-

Reference: Bachert C et al. [26].

Table 2.
Biologics selection of each characteristic pattern.

This study proved that omalizumab treatment group had clinically significant improvement with reducing the nasal polyp size.

7.3 IL-4 receptor alpha targeting agent

A first study related to dupilumab was published in the United States and Europe in the years 2013/2014. The study design was randomized, double-blind, placebo-controlled design. Total participated patients were 60, 30 refractory CRSwNP to intranasal corticosteroids plus dupilumab (a 600-mg loading dose followed by 300 mg weekly) and 30 placebo control group did this study design protocol. Treatment response comparison of two groups is demonstrated by nasal polyp score, Lund-Mackay CT total score SNOT-22, and smell function test (UPSIT). During the study, adverse effects were revealed. Nasopharyngitis (33% with placebo, 47% with dupilumab), injection site reactions (7% vs. 40%), and headache (17% vs. 20%) were presented. According to many kinds of literature, it is an effective treatment that topical steroid treatment with blocking a type 2 immune response such as antagonizing IL-4 and IL-13 controls CRSwNP.

8. Clinical application of biologics

The positive effect of biologics is revealed by many literature. Despite a lot of merits of biologics, there are some limitations of clinical application in the real world. First, high price of biologics appliance is a burden for CRSwNP patients. Sustainable biologics injection without follow-up loss is another burden. Appropriate selection of type 2 immune disease-CRSwNP patient is the other

mAbs	Mechanism of action	Dose adult (>12 years)	Mode of application
Omalizumab	Binds free IgE	75-600 mg (1–4 doses) every 2 or 4 weeks Determined by basal IgE levels, measured before starting treatment, and body weight(kg)	Subcutaneous: upper arm, thigh, or abdomen 75 mg or 150 mg powder and solvent for solution for injection. The reconstituted solution must be used immediately.
Dupilumab	Blocks IL-4Rα receptor	300 mg every 2 weeks	Subcutaneous: upper arm, thigh, or abdomen 300 mg pre-filled syringe. Store in a refrigerator (2–8°C). Do not freeze. Do not shake.
Mepolizumab	Inhibits IL-5	100 mg every 4 weeks	Subcutaneous: upper arm, thigh, or abdomen 100 mg powder to be reconstituted with 1.2 ml of water for injections. The reconstituted solution must be used immediately.
Benralizumab	Inhibits binding of IL-5 to IL-5Rα receptor Direct eosinophil cytotoxic effects	300 mg every 4 weeks for three times, and then 30 mg every 8 weeks	Subcutaneous: upper arm, thigh, or abdomen 30 mg pre-filled syringe. Store in a refrigerator (2–8°C). Do not freeze. Do not shake.
Reslizumab	Inhibits IL-5	3 mg/kg every 4 weeks	Intravenous infusion of 20–50 min through a sterile, non-pyrogenic, single use, low protein-binding infusion filter (0.2 μm). 2.5-ml or 10-ml vial. 1 ml contains 10 mg of reslizumab. Store in a refrigerator (2–8°C). Do not freeze.

Reference: Zhang and Bachert [9].

Table 3.
Biologics and biologics protocol.

consideration to attain the optimal effect. There are still debating points whether biologics treatment could be started before or after surgical approach. EPOS2020 recommended the use of biologics in the treatment of CRSwNP to improve QOL and prevent polyposis progression. Until now, there are no certain markers to predict treatment responses for biologics. According to published literature, there is no definitely predictive characteristic to evaluate the biologics treatment. Therefore, recent papers checked data after a biologics use. One of the most believable values is the recovery of the olfactory function after treatment. There are some evaluations of olfactory function such as the Sniffin' Sticks test and SNOT-22. Efficacy of dupilumab is usually checked by an evaluation of nasal polyp size, olfaction, and symptom clearance at weeks 24 and 52 after biologics treatment. Following this topic, there are summaries of biologics application and side effects in the following paragraphs [9, 31] (**Table 3** and **4**). Papacharalampous GX et al. [32] reviewed about the comparison of omalizumab, dupilumab, and mepolizumab's efficacy. In the aspects of treatment impact on nasal polyp score and sense of smell, dupilumab was the most effective agent. A recent paper reported the safety of biologics for atopic diseases during pregnancy [33]. This literature reviewed seven cases evaluating the consequences in seven women and their offspring who were exposed to

	Side effect (very common)	Side effect (common)	Very rare*
Omalizumab	Pyrexia	Headache, injection site reactions, upper abdominal pain	Allergic granulomatous vasculitis (i.e., Churg-Strauss syndrome) Alopecia, arthralgia, idiopathic thrombocytopenia Joint swelling, myalgia Serum sickness
Mepolizumab	Headache	Back pain, eczema, hypersensitivity reaction, injection site reactions, lower respiratory tract infection	-
Dupilumab	Injection site reactions	Blepharitis, conjunctivitis, hypereosinophilia, eye pruritus, headache, oral herpes	Serum sickness
Benralizumab	-	Headache, hypersensitivity reactions, injection site reactions, pharyngitis, pyrexia	Anaphylactic reaction
Reslizumab	-	Blood creatine phosphokinase increased	-

Reference: Dorling et al. [31] and Zhang and Bachert [9].

Table 4.
Biologics side effects.

dupilumab during pregnancy. According to this study, there were seven live births and one premature birth. Other literatures showed that paternal use of dupilumab does not affect male fertility and fetal outcomes [34]. In 2023, EPOS and EUFOREA progressed the evaluation of pregnant women biologics use and the change of biologics treatment (**Table 5**). Rosso C et al. present that the best fits with each biologic are mandatory to personalize the therapy [35]. Dupilumab is the most effective agent for type 2 CRSwNP, at present. In many cases of dupilumab as the first-line treatment for

Topic	Content
1. What biologics can be given to a pregnant woman?	Omalizumab is the only biologic until now that showed no increase in congenital anomalies or adverse outcomes in a registry of pregnant asthmatics treated with omalizumab.
2. Can biologics work preventively?	There are no data suggesting that biologics can prevent CRS.
3. Parameters to evaluate the "success" of biologics	Patient reported outcomes: SNOT-22, smell loss, congestion scores, comorbidities. •NP score, CT scan scores, smell tests.
4. Follow-up period to check the response of CRSwNP	Expert board advises 16 weeks to be adjusted to 6 months. After 1 year, a second evaluation is necessary, and thereafter a yearly evaluation will suffice.
5. Reasons to decrease/stop biologics	Side effects are seldom a reason to stop treatment with biologics.

Reference: Fokkens WJ et al. [34].

Table 5.
Updated information on indication and evaluation of biologics in CRSwNP according to EPOS/EUFOREA.

CRSwNP, there is a high rate of adverse effects, particularly hyper-eosinophilia. In an occurrence case of hyper-eosinophilia using dupilumab, a recommendation should be made to change to another biologic agent, especially omalizumab.

Author details

Joon Kon Kim[1,2]

1 Department of Otorhinolaryngology, Eulji University College of Medicine, Daejeon, South Korea

2 Department of Otorhinolaryngology-Head and Neck surgery, Seoul National University of College of Medicine, Seoul, South Korea

*Address all correspondence to: konddang@icloud.com

References

[1] Bachert C, Marple B, Schlosser RJ, Hopkins C, Schleimer RP, Lambrecht BN, et al. Adult chronic rhinosinusitis. Nature Reviews. Disease Primers. 2020;**6**(1):86

[2] Cergan R, Berghi ON, Dumitru M, Vrinceanu D, Manol F, Serboiu CS. Biologics for chronic rhinosinusitis-a modern option for therapy. Life. 2023;**13**:2165

[3] Kato A, Peters AT, Stevens WW, Schleimer RP, Tan BK, Kern RC. Endotypes of chronic rhinosinusitis: Relationships to disease phenotypes pathogenesis, clinical finding, and treatment approaches. Allergy. 2022;**77**(3):812-826

[4] Kim SD, Cho KS. Treatment strategy of uncontrolled chronic rhinosinusitis with nasal polyps: A review of recent evidence. International Journal of Molecular Sciences. 2023;**24**(5):5015

[5] Xu Z, Huang Y, Meese T, Van Nevel S, Holtappels G, Vanhee S, et al. The multi-omics single-cell landscape of sinus mucosa in uncontrolled severe chronic rhinosinusitis with nasal polyps. Clinical Immunology. 2023;**256**:109791

[6] Fokken WJ, Lund VJ, Mullol J, Bachert C, Alobid I, Baroody F, et al. EPOS 2012: European position paper on rhinosinusitis and nasal polyps 2012. A summary for otorhinolaryngologists. Rhinology. 2012;**50**(1):1-12

[7] Stevens WW, Peters AT, Hirsch AG, Nordberg CM, Schwartz BS, Mercer DG, et al. Clinical characteristics of patients with chronic rhinosinusitis with nasal polyps, asthma and aspirin-exacerbated respiratory disease. The Journal of Allergy and Clinical Immunology. In Practice. 2017;**5**(4):1061-70.e3

[8] Jenkins C, Costello J, Hodge L. Systematic review of prevalence of aspirin induced asthma and its implications for clinical practice. BMJ. 2004;**328**(7437):434

[9] Zhang L, Bachert C, editors. Chronic Rhinosinusitis. Singapore: Springer Nature; 2022

[10] Mascia K, Haselkorn T, Deniz YM, Miller DP, Bleecker ER, Borish L, et al. Aspirin sensitivity and severity of asthma: Evidence for irreversible airway obstruction in patients with severe or difficult-to-treat asthma. The Journal of Allergy and Clinical Immunology. 2005;**116**(5):970-975

[11] Wise SK, Ghegan MD, Gorham E, Schlosser RJ. Socioeconomic factors in the diagnosis of allergic fungal rhinosinusitis. Otolaryngology and Head and Neck Surgery. 2008;**138**(1):38-42

[12] Bent JP III, Kuhn FA. Diagnosis of allergic fungal sinusitis. Otolaryngology and Head and Neck Surgery. 1994;**111**(5):580-588

[13] Groh M, Pagnoux C, Baldini C, Bel E, Bottero P, Cottin V, et al. Eosinophilic granulomatosis with polyangiitis (Churg-Strauss) (EGPA) consensus task force recommendations for evaluation and management. European Journal of Internal Medicine. 2015;**26**(7):545-553

[14] Stammberger H, Posawetz W. Functional endoscopic sinus surgery. Concept, indications and results of the Messerklinger technique. European Archives of Oto-Rhino-Laryngology. 1990;**247**(2):63-76

[15] Bassiouni A, Wormald PJ. Role of frontal sinus surgery in nasal

polyp recurrence. Laryngoscope. 2013;**123**(1):36-41

[16] Soyka MB, Wawrzyniak P, Eiwegger T, Holzmann D, Treis A, Wanke K, et al. Defective epithelial barrier in chronic rhinosinusitis: The regulation of tight junctions by IFN-γ and IL-4. The Journal of Allergy and Clinical Immunology. 2012;**130**(5):1087-96.e10

[17] Rimmer J, Fokkens W, Chung LY, Hoplins C. Surgical versus medical interventions for chronic rhinosinusitis with nasal polyps. Cochrane Database of Systematic Reviews. 2014;2014(12):CD006991

[18] Vlaminck S, Vauterin T, Hellings PW, Jorissen M, Acke F, Van Cauwenberge P, et al. The importance of local eosinophilia in the surgical outcome of chronic rhinosinusitis: A 3-year prospective observational study. American Journal of Rhinology & Allergy. 2014;**28**(3):260-264

[19] Soler ZM, Sauer DA, Mace J, Smith TL. Relationship between clinical measures and histopathologic findings in chronic rhinosinusitis. Otolaryngology and Head and Neck Surgery. 2009;**141**(4):454-461

[20] Tokunaga T, Sakashita M, Haruna T, Asaka D, Takeno S, Ikeda H, et al. Novel scoring system and algorithm for classifying chronic rhinosinusitis: The JESREC study. Allergy. 2015;**70**(8):995-1003

[21] Ikeda K, Shiozawa A, Ono N, Kusunoki T, Hirotsu M, Homma H, et al. Subclassification of chronic rhinosinusitis with nasal polyp based on eosinophil and neutrophil. Laryngoscope. 2013;**123**(11):E1-E9

[22] Matsuwaki Y, Ookushi T, Asaka D, Mori E, Nakajima T, Yoshida T, et al. Chronic rhinosinusitis: Risk factors for the recurrence of chronic rhinosinusitis based on 5-year follow-up after endoscipic sinus surgery. International Archives of Allergy and Immunology. 2008;**146**(Suppl. 1):77-81

[23] Meng Y, Zhang L, Lou H, Wang C. Predictive value of computed tomography in the recurrence of chronic rhinosinusitis with nasal polyps. International Forum of Allergy & Rhinology. 2019;**9**(11):1236-1243

[24] Gevaert P, Calus L, Van Zele T, Blomme K, De Ruyck N, Bauters W, et al. Omalizumab is effective in allergic and nonallergic patients with nasal polyps and asthma. The Journal of Allergy and Clinical Immunology. 2013;**131**(1):110-116

[25] Bachert C, Han JK, Desrosiers M, Hellings PW, Amin N, Lee SE, et al. Efficacy and safety of dupilumab in patients with severe chronic rhinosinusitis with nasal polyps (LIBERTY NP SINUS-24 and LIBERTY NP SINUS-52): Results from two multi-Centre, randomized, double-blind, placebo-controlled, parallel-group phase 3 trials. Lancet (London). 2019;**394**(10209):1638-1650

[26] Bachert C et al. The Journal of Allergy and Clinical Immunology. 2018;**141**(5):1543-1551

[27] Jonstam K, Swanson BN, Mannent LP, Cardell LO, Tian N, Wang Y, et al. Dupilumab reduces local type 2 pro-inflammatory biomarkers in chronic rhinosinusitis with nasal polyposis. Allergy. 2019;**74**(4):743-752

[28] Corren J. New targeted therapies for uncontrolled asthma. The Journal of Allergy and Clinical Immunology. In Practice. 2019;7(5):1394-1403

[29] Dávila González I, Moreno Benítez F, Quirce S. Benralizumab: A new approach for the treatment of severe eosinophilic asthma. Journal of Investigational Allergology & Clinical Immunology. 2019;**29**(2):84-93

[30] Zhang N, Holtappels G, Gevaert P, Patuou J, Dhaliwal B, Gould H, et al. Mucosal tissue polyclonal IgE is functional in response to allergen and SEB. Allergy. 2011;**66**(1):141-148

[31] Dorling M, Hernaiz-Leonardo JC, Pascual A, Janjua A, Thamboo A, Javer A. Real-world adverse events after type 2 biologic use in chronic rhinosinusitis with nasal polyps. Laryngoscope. 2024;**134**:3054-3059

[32] Papacharalampous GX, Constantinidis J, Fotiadis G, Zhang N, Bachert C, Katotomichelakis M. Chronic rhinosinusitis with nasal polyps (CRSwNP) treated with omalizumab, dupilumab, or mepolizumab: A systematic review of the current knowledge towards an attempt to compare agents' efficacy. International Forum of Allergy & Rhinology. 2024;**14**:96-109

[33] Shakuntulla F, Chiarella SE. Safety of biologics for atopic diseases during pregnancy. The Journal of Allergy and Clinical Immunology. In Practice. 2022;**10**(12):3149-3155

[34] Fokkens WJ, Viskens AS, Backer V, Conti D, Corso E, Gevaert P, et al. EPOS/EUFOREA update on indication and evaluation of biologics in chronic rhinosinusitis with nasal polyps 2023. Rhinology. 2023;**61**(3):194-202

[35] Rosso C, Corso ED, Conti V, Nitro L, Saibene AM, Parazzini E, et al. Switching of biological therapy to dupilumab in comorbid patients with severe asthma and CRSwNP. European Archives of Oto-Rhino-Laryngology. 2024;**281**(6):3017-3023

Chapter 7

Vibrant Soundbridge Surgical Techniques

Isra Aljazeeri, Anas Ibrahim, Yassin Abdelsamad and Farid Alzhrani

Abstract

The Vibrant Soundbridge device is an active middle ear implant that converts the acoustic energy to a vibratory signal that is delivered to the middle ear. Along with bypassing the conductive element of hearing process lateral to the side of attachment, the VSB can also give some amplification to the hearing. The VSB was first FDA approved for treating patients with SNHL, and now the candidacy expanded to cover patients with mixed and pure conductive hearing loss and has proven its success in practice. The device consists of an external speech processor with a microphone that receives the sound and an internal part with an internal receiver coil, a conductor link, and a floating mass transducer (FMT). The vibrating part of the VSB is the FMT, which is coupled to the ossicular chain using various vibroplasty couplers to fit a wide variety of anatomical differences of the patients.

Keywords: otology, neurotology, surgery, surgical techniques, middle ear implant, implantable device, vibrant Soundbridge, conductive hearing loss, sensorineural hearing loss

1. Introduction

The Vibrant Soundbridge device is an active middle ear implant that converts the acoustic energy to a vibratory signal to be delivered to the middle ear. This implantable device is intended for patients who cannot benefit from the conventional hearing aids. Along with bypassing the conductive element of hearing process lateral to the side of attachment, the VSB can also give some amplification to the hearing. The VSB was first FDA approved for treating patients with SNHL and now the candidacy expanded to cover patients with mixed and pure conductive hearing loss and has proven its success in practice.

2. Device

The device consists of an external audio processor (AP) with a microphone that receives the sound and an internal part named VORP. The skin over the internal part

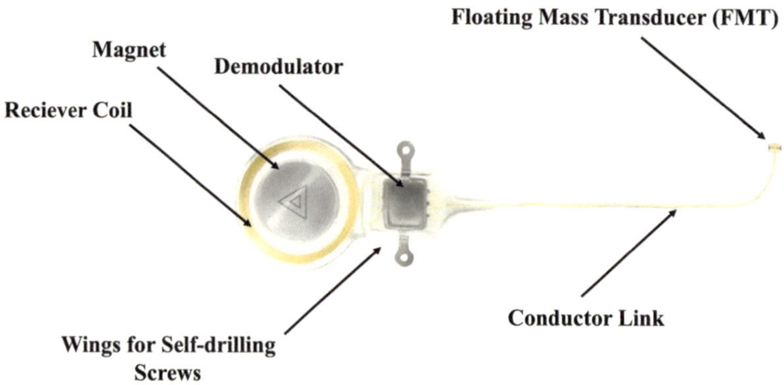

Figure 1.
Illustration of the VORP, which is the internal part of the Vibrant Soundbridge, surgically implanted.

of the implant stays intact after implantation, avoiding the skin complications of percutaneous implantation. The AP is kept in place over the scalp via magnet connection to the internal part, without the need to be hanged over an auricle that might be missing or malformed in some patients. The energy source for the device is a battery installed inside the AP in the outer part. There are two microphones in the AP providing some directional element to the hearing.

The VORP consists of an internal receiver coil surrounding a magnet, a modulator, fixation wings, a conductor link, and a floating mass transducer (FMT) (**Figure 1**). The fixation wings of the VORP are fixed to the skull using two self-drilling screws. The vibrating part of the VSB is the FMT, which is coupled to the ossicular chain using various vibroplasty couplers to fit a wide variety of anatomical differences of the patients. The FMT should be attached only to a single middle ear structure without touching any other surrounding temporal bone. This allows for free mobility of the FMT. Additionally, the growth of the skull will not affect the position of the FMT, making it suitable for use in pediatric patients.

3. Preoperative imaging

Studying the preoperative CT of the temporal bone can help the surgical planning for VSB implantation. Using the Burd et al. preoperative imagining checklist is advisable to evaluate for the anatomical parameters of the surgical access, the attachment sites, and the limitations to the surgery [1].

In case of congenital aural atresia, Frenzel et al. CT-based scoring system is helpful for precise risk stratification prior to VSB surgery [2].

4. Surgical approach

Surgical application of VSB is a very delicate surgery. It is possible that due to intraoperative findings or difficulties, the application of VSB would not be possible. For this reason, in cases with conductive hearing loss, where the candidacy allows, a back-up bone conductive device should be available, and the patient should be consented for this possibility. Furthermore, the site of the coupling, although can be predicted by studying the preoperative CT, is ultimately decided upon the intraoperative status of the middle ear.

4.1 Incision

4.1.1 Standard incision

The incision for VSB can be the same postauricular incision as with cortical mastoidectomy, placed about 5 mm behind the postauricular sulcus, extending from 1 cm above the mastoid tip for 3 cm (**Figure 2**).

Then, the skin is pulled outwards to help identify the superior periosteum that does not get retracted and is stuck to the skull bone. This level is the level of the first layer incision. Undermining at this level is very smooth and effortless superiorly, and then, it has to extend anteriorly to the level of the EAC and superior–anteriorly to the level of expected zygomatic arch. Posterior undermining should be done to prevent tension upon skin closure. Inferior undermining should be done with care not to extend beyond the mastoid tip to avoid FN injury.

The second layer of the incision is the periosteal flap that can be either done as an anterior-based palva flap, T-shaped flap, or superior-based flap. Either of these flaps can achieve the exposure needed for the mastoidectomy.

4.1.2 Modified incision

There is a large proportion of VSB candidates who have auricular deformities like microtia and anotia. These patients might need future reconstructive surgeries, for which local flaps might be needed. The superficial temporal artery (STA) and its

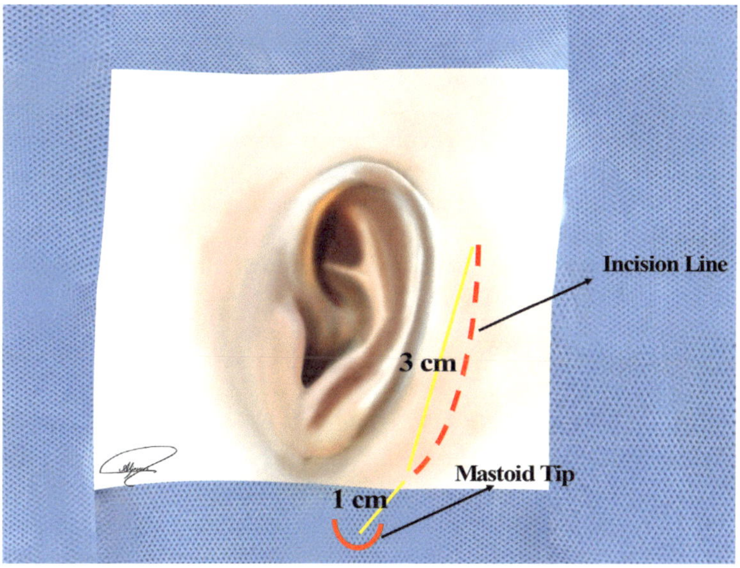

Figure 2.
Incision line in cases with normal auricle is the same as standard mastoidectomy incision. About 5 mm to 1 cm behind the postauricular sulcus, 1 cm above the mastoid tip and of 3 cm length.

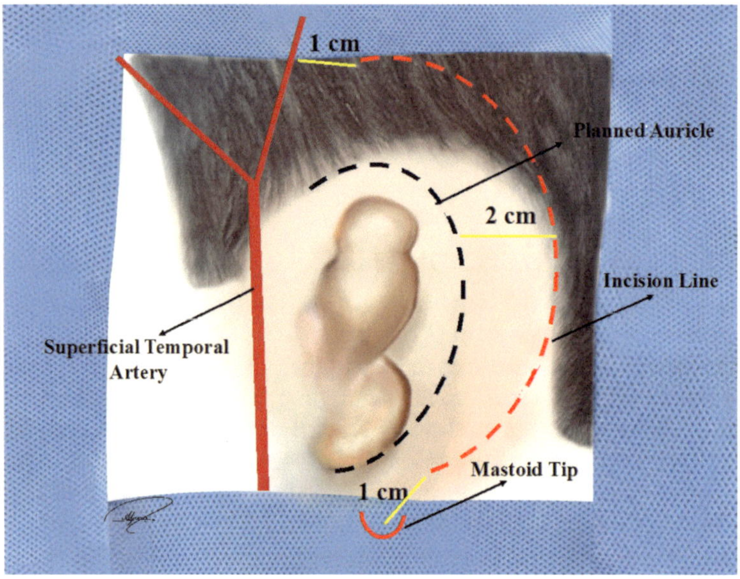

Figure 3.
In cases of anotia and microtia, a modified incision is used. First, the surgeon marks the area of planned reconstruction of the auricle and marks the superior temporal artery that is located by palpation. The modified incision is starting 1 cm above the mastoid tip and running 2 cm behind the planned auricle line. This incision should stop at least 1 cm behind the posterior branch of the STA.

branches are the feeding arteries for multiple local flaps that can be used for auricular reconstruction and thus need to be preserved during VSB implantation surgeries. A modified incision should be used in these cases [3].

The surgeon needs to palpate for the site of the STA, and the incision should end 1 cm before the area of the STA. Furthermore, the incision in these cases needs to avoid the area of the planned auricle. The planned auricle should be marked first, assuming the normal size of an adult-sized full auricle, ranging from 5.5 to 6.5 cm in height, with a width of ½ to 1/3rd of its height [4].

The surgical incision for VSB should be at least 2 cm behind the level of the planned auricle to avoid having the scar at the site of reconstruction. The modified incision should be done in one layer, directly to the bone level. The skin and the periosteum should be elevated together without separation from each other. The anterior limit of the flap elevation anteriorly is to the level of the TMJ since there is no EAC. The periosteum at the site of the TMJ converges inward, providing a view very similar to what happens with the EAC (**Figure 3**).

4.2 Skin flap

A sub-periosteal pocket for the VORP 503 is then created by posterior–superior elevation of the periosteum from the skull. This can be done using a freer elevator, facing the bone, in a fan-shaped rotation movement (**Figure 4**).

The VORP 503 template is used to ensure the pocket has an appropriate size. The skin flap over the magnet should not exceed 7 mm to ensure coupling of the magnet to the sound processor. This can be done using the Skin Flap Gauge 7. Alternatively, the measurement can be done directly by inserting a needle perpendicularly into the sterile skin and measuring the inserted depth. This is optimally

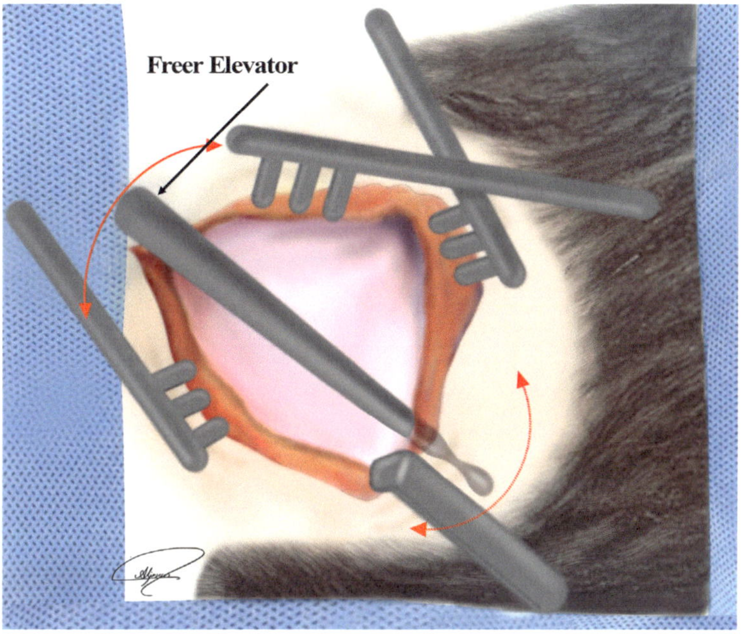

Figure 4.
Sub-periosteal pocket for the VORP is made by elevation of the periosteum from the skull using freer elevator in a fan-shaped rotational movement.

should be done before injecting the area with local analgesic solution to avoid over estimation.

In the case that the skin flap is thicker than 7 mm, thinning should be done with caution. Overthinning can lead to flap necrosis at the site of the magnet. This can be done using a blunt tip scissor in a dissecting motion and not a cutting motion, to create a new pocket in a level suspected to give a lateral thickness of 7 mm. After which, the medial portion can be cut.

4.3 Mastoidectomy

Cortical mastoidectomy should be done widely (**Figure 5**). Removing the cells along the tegmen helps widening the antrum and aditus to allow maximum space for coupling the FMT on the short process.

While removing the cells along the sinodural angle helps identifying the area where the VORP 503 demodulator should be placed outside the mastoid air cell system, in a compact cortical bone. The demodulator template can be used at this stage to make a transitional tunnel with or without a bony bridge cover at the lateral end of the sinodural angle (**Figure 6**).

Further steps depend on the type of the coupler that is planned to be used. Any coupler other than the short processor coupler will need facial recess approach and might need elevation of the tympanomeatal flap to widen the exposure.

An important note is that the ossicles are extremely delicate and can easily be eroded or dislocated using a cutting bur or by any manipulations. Using a diamond burr, a wide exposure and careful handling the instrument near the ossicles is advised. The surgeon's hand needs to be supported to avoid any jerky unplanned movements.

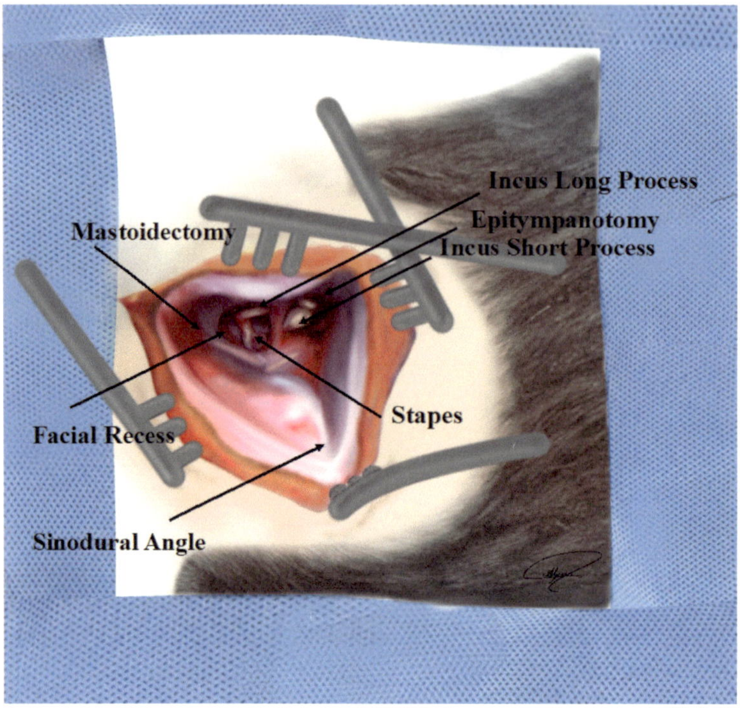

Figure 5.
Anatomical landmarks seen after mastoidectomy.

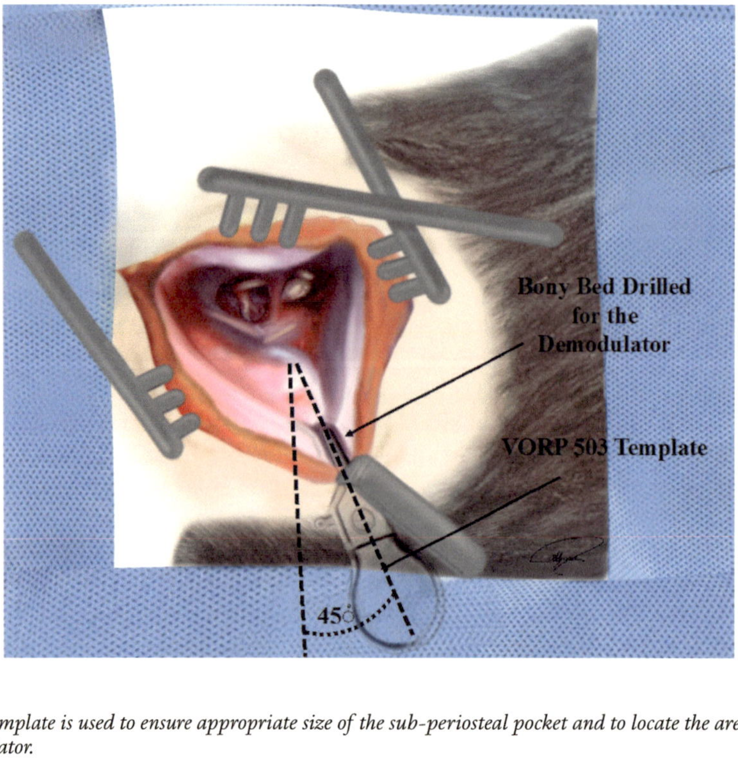

Figure 6.
VORP 502 template is used to ensure appropriate size of the sub-periosteal pocket and to locate the area to drill for the demodulator.

4.3.1 Posterior epitympanotomy

The incus short process can be exposed through posterior epitympanotomy to apply an incus-SP coupler. The incus short process coupler use was first described (**Figure 7**) by Farid et al. [5].

This approach needs an intact and mobile ossicular chain medial to the incus in cases with pure sensorineural hearing loss. However, examination of the mobility of the incus is crucial when this approach is used in cases of ossicular malformations that happen in association with microtia.

To apply the incus-SP coupler an appropriate space is needed in the attic area superior to the incus. Thus, it is important to properly skeletonize the tegmen with particular attention, not to touch the incus while drilling. It is advisable to use small diameter diamond bur, while keeping all the edges of the bur visible at all times. The FMT sizer then can be used to evaluate the planned placement area. The lateral and media borders of the short process are then checked with a thin tipped instrument like a needle to make sure there is enough space for the coupling clips and there are no adhesions to the walls.

In cases of aural atresia, there is a possibility of anomalies in the short process of the incus. If the surgeon is of any doubt of fixation of the incus due to these anomalies, it is advised to open the facial recess and examine the mobility of the ossicular chain.

4.3.2 Facial recess approach

Through a facial recess approach, it is possible to couple the incus-LP, vibroplasty-clip, and RW-soft couplers or to perform direct FMT to RW coupling. For cases where incus-LP coupling is intended, anterior and superior widening of the facial recess will allow for full visualization of the long process of the incus (**Figures 8** and **9**).

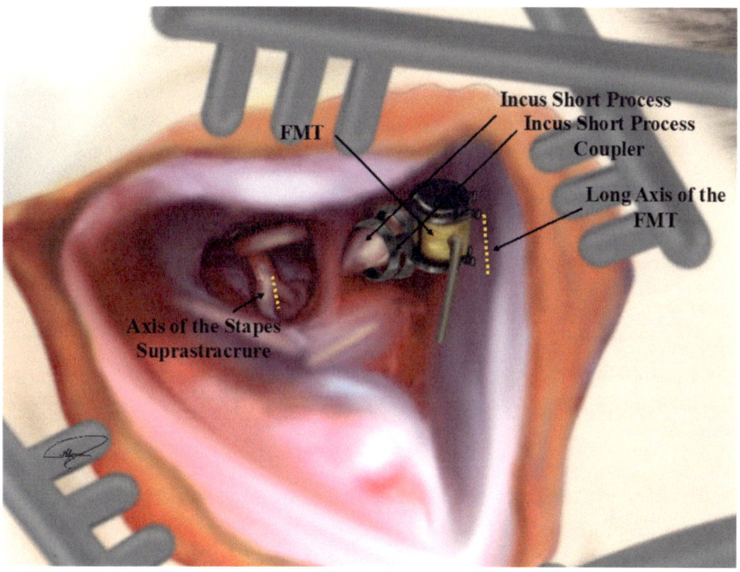

Figure 7.
Illustration of an FMT coupled using incus short process coupler. The long axis of the FMT should be parallel to the axis of the stapes suprastructure.

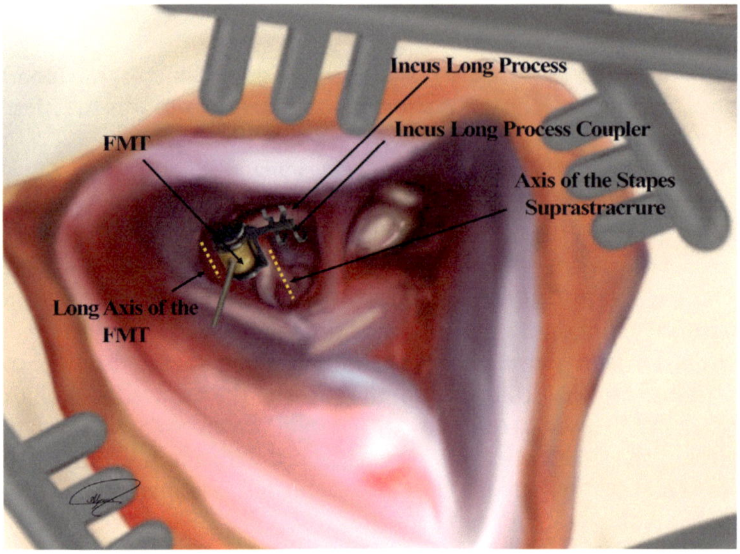

Figure 8.
Illustration of an FMT coupled using incus long process coupler. The long axis of the FMT should be parallel to the axis of the stapes suprastructure.

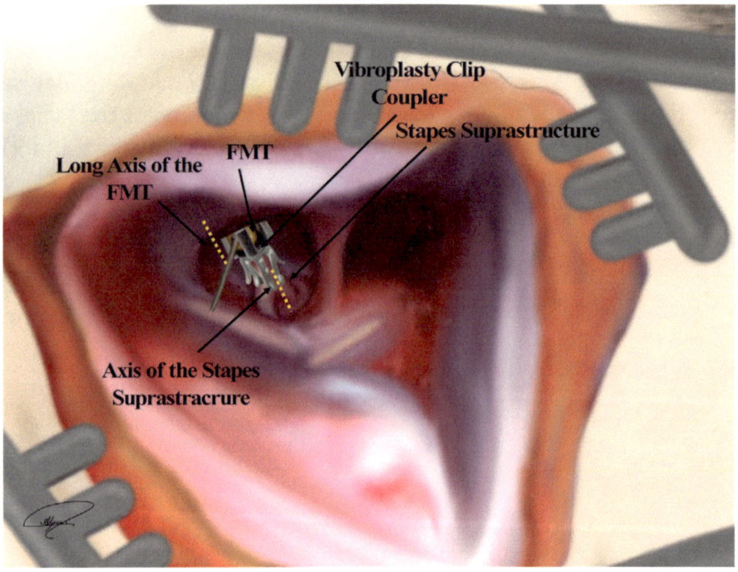

Figure 9.
Illustration of an FMT coupled using stapes coupler. The long axis of the FMT should be parallel to the axis of the stapes suprastructure.

A minimum of a 3 mm facial recess width will be required to allow for the passage of a 2.3 mm long FMT along with its coupler. In some cases, the facial recess may be too narrow that it barely allows the passage of the FMT with the coupler, making surgical manipulation and mounting difficult due to the poor visualization. In these cases, elevation of the tympanomeatal flap can increase the window of visualization through the transcanal approach.

Patients with aural atresia are at higher risk of anomalous course of facial nerve. Proper preoperative study of the CT and the use of intraoperative facial nerve monitor is of utmost importance.

4.4 RW vibroplasty

In cases where RW vibroplasty is planned, there is a risk of puncturing the RWM during drilling of the RWN (**Figures 10** and **11**). To prevent SNHL, it is advised to prepare a piece of fascia or perichondrium prior to drilling to immediately seal the RW in cases of endolymph leak. Suctioning the endolymph will also increase the risk of SNHL and must be avoided [6].

4.5 Radical cavity

One of the indications of VSB implantation is the CHL and MHL in patients with radical cavity post canal wall down mastoidectomy. In some cases, these patients lack any remnants of ossicular chain to which the coupler is usually attached. The option for these patients is to do round window vibroplasty in which the FMT is connected to the round window (**Figure 12**).

It is of crucial importance to remove all the epithelial tissue over the middle ear and the cavity to prevent later development of cholesteatoma. Then the area of the RW is identified and all the fibrosis and adhesions are removed. To expose the RW membrane, the bony overhanging niche should be drilled. Care must be taken not to penetrate the RW membrane.

Next, the FMT sizer can help identify any site of overhanging bony protuberances that need to be drilled. The axis of the FMT needs to be perpendicular to the round window membrane. The surgeon can either use autologous soft tissue interface between the FMT and the RW or use a RW-soft coupler. Then the FMT needs to be

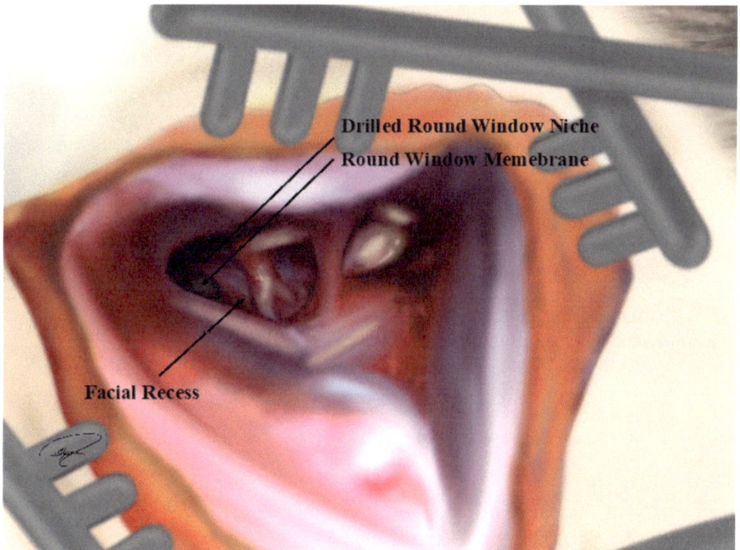

Figure 10.
Illustration of the anatomical position of the round window vibroplasty.

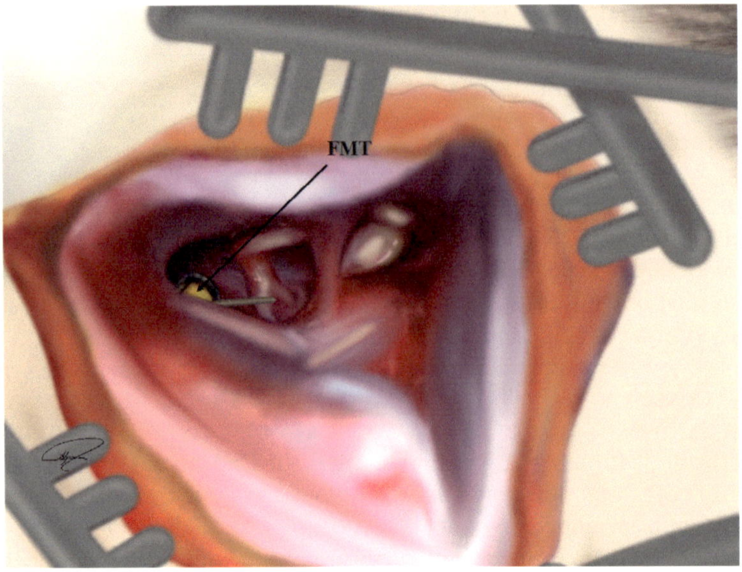

Figure 11.
Illustration of an FMT coupled to the round window membrane. The long axis of the FMT should be perpendicular to the round window membrane.

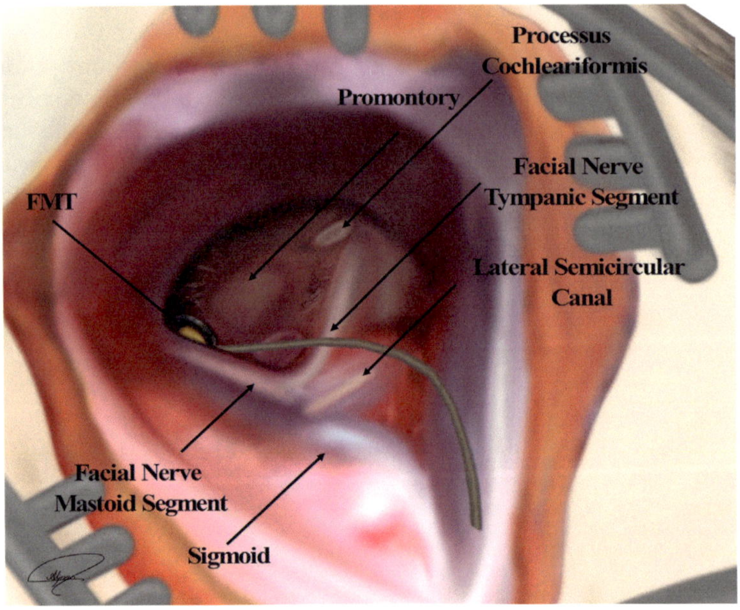

Figure 12.
Illustration of an FMT coupled to the round window membrane in a canal wall down mastoid cavity.

fixed in place by packing the gap between inferior face and the bony hypotympanum using cartilage pieces.

A high jugular bulb can limit the inferior boundary for the FMT placement. Careful study of the preoperative CT is thus of importance to know this limitation. In case of inadvertent jugular bleeding, direct pressure and waiting for about 15 minutes

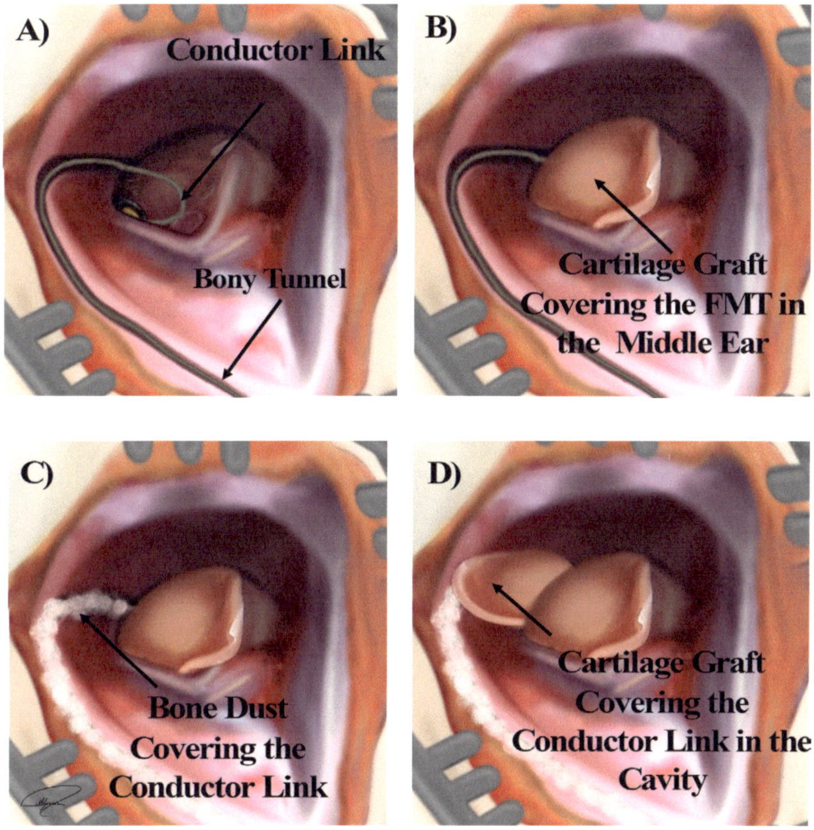

Figure 13.
Illustrating the steps for stabilization of the device in canal wall down mastoid cavities. (A) A bony bed is drilled inferiorly, anterior to the location of the facial nerve, directing the conductor link from the middle ear, laterally, toward the outer skull cortex. (B) The FMT in the middle ear is covered with a piece of cartilage graft. The edges of this cartilage graft are inserted underneath the medial bony edges of the facial recess and the anterior canal wall. (C) The conductor link in the bony tunnel is covered with bone dust. (D) The bony tunnel in the mastoid cavity is covered by pieces of cartilage grafts.

can help stop the bleeding. In these cases, it is an option to couple the FMT to the oval window instead. This is a challenging option since the lateral support for fixation of the FMT will be missing. A cartilage tympanoplasty can be used, which is not as reliable as a RW vibroplasty.

In cases with radical cavity, a proper cartilaginous coverage for the conductor link will be needed to prevent risk of device extrusion. The conductor link should lie closest to the bony bed, with no right angulations, and covered entirely with pieces of cartilage. A sheet of bone dust over the conductor link in the mastoid cavity and away from the FMT area can also be used for long term fixation (**Figure 13**). But this technique can put the link at higher risk of breakage in case a revision surgery is needed. An alternative technique to this cartilaginous coverage is to perform blind sac closure.

4.6 Controlled movement technique

For the application of the coupler to the ossicles, there is an amount of force that needs to be applied to the coupler. Due to the delicate nature of the ossicles, applying this force can lead to ossicular dislocation. The other consideration is that the claws of the coupler need to spread before hugging the ossicle. The force directed to the coupler aiming to spread its claws can lead to slipping of the coupler away without getting coupled.

To solve these two issues that can be frustrating to the surgeon, a "controlled" movement technique is suggested. In this technique, two instruments should be used: one exerting the main force and one controlling the direction of the main force.

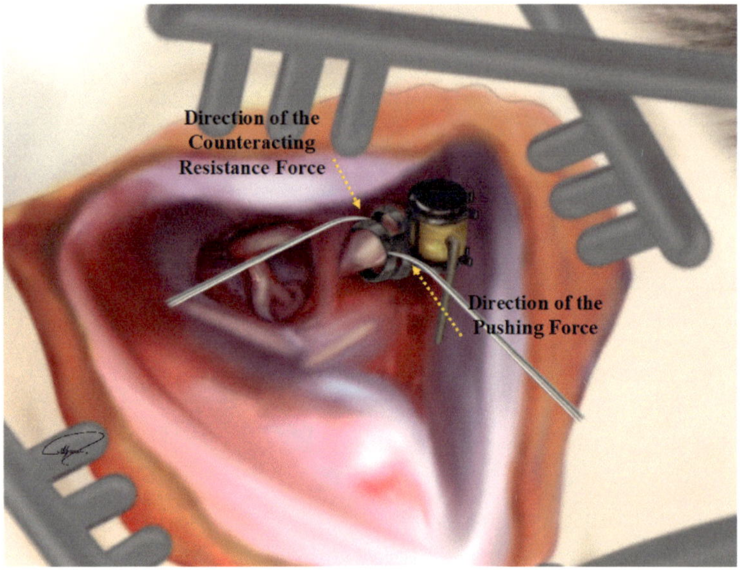

Figure 14.
Illustration of the controlled movement technique while mounting the incus short process coupler.

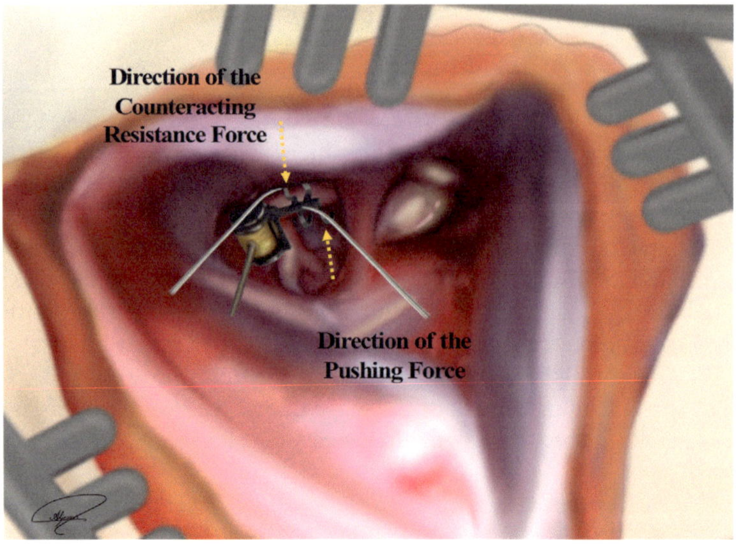

Figure 15.
Illustration of the controlled movement technique while mounting the incus long process coupler.

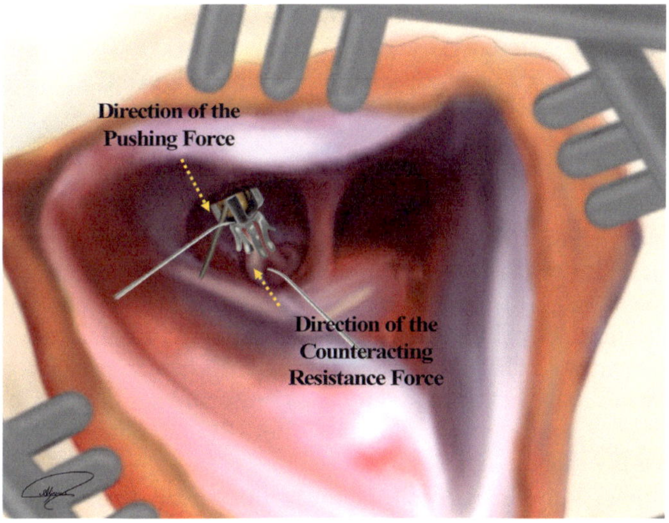

Figure 16.
Illustration of the controlled movement technique while mounting the stapes coupler.

The controlling instrument should be placed behind the ossicle without moving to support the ossicle from being dislocated. And it can be used against the direction where the coupler slips to correct the trajectory of movement (**Figures 14–16**).

4.7 Post-mastoidectomy depression

After doing cortical mastoidectomy, a bony defect will develop that can inadvertently affect the site of auricular reconstruction in cases of auricular deformity. In these cases, reconstructing this defect can help the esthetic appearance. This can be

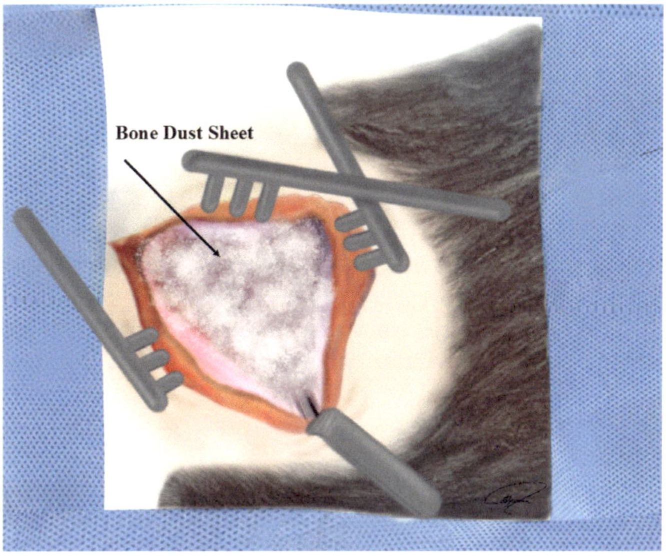

Figure 17.
Illustration of post-mastoidectomy covered with a bone dust sheet.

done by the bony pate of the mastoidectomy. The bone pate can be collected in a dry container, till the end of the surgery. Then it can be pressed as a sheet and be used to replace the cortical bone of the mastoidectomy cavity (**Figure 17**).

5. Complications

The possible complications of doing VSB surgery can be divided into approach-related complications and the complications of the device. The approach-related complications are similar to mastoidectomy, due to the surgical instrumentation close to anatomical structures including bleeding, taste disturbance, facial nerve paralysis, CSF leak, and vertigo. Additionally, when the ossicles are manipulated, there is risk for additional conductive hearing loss and even sensorineural hearing loss. The opening of the round window membrane in cases where RW coupling is performed may lead to deafness if endolymph leak happens.

Device complications include device failure, incomplete gap closure, flap necrosis, and conductor link extrusion in cavities.

There is also a risk for general complications like chronic pain and postoperative surgical site infection which can endanger the soiling of the implant and necessitate explanation.

6. Intraoperative testing

For the VSB to be able to deliver the sound in an efficient manner, it needs proper coupling. This includes appropriate direction of the long axis of the FMT, which needs to be parallel to the direction of the stapes suprastructure in incus-SP, incus-LP, clip, and OW couplers. And it should be perpendicular to the RWM in cases of RW vibroplasty. These orientations of the FMT allow for the maximum vibrating energy being directed to the inner ear and avoiding loss of energy in a direction that does not result in hearing.

Furthermore, the FMT and its coupled middle ear structure need to be freely mobile to be able to vibrate.

It is particularly more difficult to evaluate proper coupling in cases with RW coupling. This is because the FMT needs to be pressed enough against the RWM in a degree that allows for vibration transmission without being loose to fall and without being over-pressed in a degree that loses possibility to vibrate. For these reasons, trials have been made to develop an objective method to evaluate intraoperative coupling to avoid revision repositioning. Various intraoperative electrical response audiometry measures have been tried, including auditory steady state response (ASSR), auditory brainstem response (ABR), and electrocochleography (ECochG) [7–15].

To get an electrical response, vibratory stimulus needs to be presented by the FMT of the VSB. This stimulus can be delivered as an auditory stimulus through the audio processor or by wireless streaming a pre-recorded signal to the audio processor. Both of these methods have inherited limitations that can affect the interpretation of the outcomes, since the signal will be modified during processing and the gain settings need to be adjusted as per the patients' hearing condition. On the other hand, the complexity of recording procedure limited the wide use of ECochG.

To overcome these limitations, AcoustiAP device has been developed. This device provides direct signal transmission from the ABR machine to the FMT that does not undergo processing. The device is compatible with most ABR machines, which have a jack socket output of 6.35 mm [16]. If intraoperative ABR is planned for the patient, the electrodes for ABR machine need to be applied before the draping of the patient to keep the sterility of the surgical field.

Conflict of interest

The author declares no conflict of interest.

Author details

Isra Aljazeeri[1,2]*, Anas Ibrahim[3], Yassin Abdelsamad[3] and Farid Alzhrani[2]

1 Aljaber Ophthalmology and Otolaryngology Hospital, Otolaryngology Department, Ministry of Health, Ahsa, Saudi Arabia

2 King Abdullah Ear Specialist Center (KAESC), College of Medicine, King Saud University Medical City (KSUMC), King Saud University, Riyadh, Saudi Arabia

3 Research Department, MED-EL GmbH, Riyadh, Saudi Arabia

*Address all correspondence to: dr.isra.aljazeeri@gmail.com

References

[1] Burd C, Pai I, Connor SE. Active middle ear implantation: Imaging in the pre-operative planning and post-operative assessment of the vibrant Soundbridge™. The British Journal of Radiology. 2020;**93**(1109):20190741

[2] Frenzel H, Sprinzl GM, Widmann G, Petersen D, Wollenberg B, Mohr C. Grading system for the selection of patients with congenital aural atresia for active middle ear implants. Neuroradiology. 2013;**55**(7):895-911

[3] Yoshimura H, Takahashi M, Iwasaki S, Shinagawa J, Takashimizu I, Nagai F, et al. Vibrant soundbridge implantation prior to auricular reconstruction with unilateral microtia-atresia. Clinical Case Reports. 2021;**9**(8):e04408

[4] Zopf DA, Knecht E, Kim JS. Microtia reconstruction. In: Cummings Pediatric Otolaryngology. 2nd ed. Facial Plastic Surgery Clinics of North America. 2021. pp. 249-258

[5] Alzhrani F, Halawani R, Yousef M. Feasibility and efficacy of vibrant Soundbridge short process coupler in patients with aural atresia. Otology & Neurotology. 2020;**41**(10):e1219-e1223

[6] Beltrame AM, Todt I, Sprinzl G, Profant M, Schwab B. Consensus statement on round window Vibroplasty. Annals of Otology, Rhinology & Laryngology. 2014;**123**(10):734-740

[7] Verhaegen V, Mulder S, Noten JFP, Luijten B, Cremers CWRJ, Snik AFM. Intraoperative auditory steady state response measurements during vibrant Soundbridge middle ear implantation in patients with mixed hearing loss. Otology Neurotology. 2010;**31**(9):1365-1368

[8] Radeloff A, Shehata-Dieler W, Rak K, Scherzed A, Tolsdorff B, Hagen R, et al. Intraoperative monitoring of active middle ear implant function in patients with Normal and pathologic middle ears. Otology & Neurotology. 2011;**32**(1):104-107

[9] Elberling C, Don M, Cebulla M, StürzebecherE. Auditory steady-state responses to chirp stimuli based on cochlear traveling wave delay. The Journal of the Acoustical Society of America. 2007;**122**(5):2772

[10] Colletti V, Mandalà M, Colletti L. Electrocochleography in round window vibrant Soundbridge implantation. Otolaryngology–Head and Neck Surgery. 2011;**146**(4):633-640

[11] Mandalà M, Colletti L, Colletti V. Treatment of the atretic ear with round window vibrant Soundbridge implantation in infants and children. Otology & Neurotology. 2011;**32**(8):1250-1255

[12] Cebulla M, Geiger U, Hagen R, Radeloff A. Device optimised chirp stimulus for ABR measurements with an active middle ear implant. International Journal of Audiology. 2017;**56**(8):607-611

[13] Geiger U, Radeloff A, Hagen R, Cebulla M. Intraoperative estimation of the coupling efficiency and clinical outcomes of the vibrant Soundbridge active middle ear implant using auditory brainstem response measurements. American Journal of Audiology. 2019;**28**(3):553-559

[14] Fröhlich L, Rahne T, Plontke SK, Oberhoffner T, Dahl R, Mlynski R, et al. Intraoperative quantification of floating mass transducer coupling quality in

active middle ear implants: A multicenter study. European Archives of Oto-Rhino-Laryngology. 2020;**278**(7):2277-2288

[15] Fröhlich L, Rahne T, Plontke SK, Oberhoffner T, Dziemba O, Gadyuchko M, et al. Intraoperative recording of auditory brainstem responses for monitoring of floating mass transducer coupling efficacy during revision surgery—Proof of concept. Otology Neurotology. 2020;**41**(2):e168-e171

[16] Sprinzl GM, Schörg P, Edlinger S, Ploder M, Magele A. Clinical feasibility of a novel test setup for objective measurements using the vibrant soundbridge. Laryngoscope Investigative Otolaryngology. 2022;7(4):1113-1119

Chapter 8

Evolution in the Treatment of Sinonasal Inverted Papillomas

Georgios Giourgos

Abstract

Sinonasal inverted papilloma is a benign neoplasm with a propensity for local invasion and potential malignant transformation. Complete surgical excision is the mainstay of treatment to prevent recurrence and the development of malignancy. Endoscopic techniques have revolutionized the surgical management of inverted papilloma, offering minimally invasive approaches with excellent visualization of the surgical field. These techniques allow for more complete resections and reduce postoperative morbidity compared to traditional open approaches. However, the complex anatomy of the paranasal sinuses and the variable extent of tumor involvement necessitate careful preoperative planning and experienced surgeons. Challenges in the management of inverted papilloma include the deep location of lesions, their tendency to infiltrate bony structures, and the potential for recurrence. The choice of surgical approach depends on the extent and location of the tumor, as well as the patient's individual characteristics. Evolution in the endoscopic techniques, with a focus on the treatment of the tumor site of origin, has emerged in most cases. More extensive tumors may require combined approaches or image-guided surgery. Preventing recurrence is a critical aspect of management. Regular follow-up with endoscopic examinations and imaging studies is essential to detect early signs of tumor regrowth. Complete removal of tumor margins is crucial to minimize the risk of recurrence.

Keywords: inverted papilloma, endoscopic surgery, paranasal sinuses, recurrence, nasal tumors

1. Introduction

Inverted papillomas (IPs) are the most common sinonasal tumors, known for their aggressive behavior, trend for recurrence, multicentricity, and potential associated malignancy. Symptoms are specific and patients typically present with unilateral nasal obstruction, discharge, epistaxis, or headache. While nasal endoscopy and imaging studies (CT, MRI) can suggest the diagnosis, histopathology is definitive. Complete surgical resection, mostly *via* a transnasal endoscopic approach, is crucial to prevent recurrence. Open or combined approaches are used in selected cases. The trend to recur is related mainly to incomplete primary resection. The extent of surgery depends on the tumor's location and size. Associated malignancies require a multidisciplinary approach and additional treatment.

2. Epidemiological data

Inverted papillomas (IP) are relatively uncommon nasal tumors, affecting approximately 0.6–1.5 people per 100,000 annually. They primarily affect adults in their 50 and 60s, with a male-to-female ratio of 2–3:1. Although IP can occur in children, it is less common. While the exact etiology remains unclear, various factors have been implicated, including chronic inflammation, viral infections (HPV, EBV), smoking, and occupational or environmental exposures [1–3].

3. Endoscopic presentation

- Polypoid mass: It often appears as a fleshy, papillomatous mass that can be sessile (attached by a broad base) or pedunculated (attached by a stalk).
- Color: Typically, it is pinkish-red, but the color can vary.
- Surface: The surface is often lobulated with a soft, friable consistency.
- Location: It can occur anywhere in the nasal cavity and paranasal sinuses but is mostly found in the middle and superior meatus.
- Extent: The extent can range from small, localized lesions to large, invasive tumors that involve multiple sinuses.

4. Radiological assessment

4.1 CT scan

Usually, the first radiological examination executed in sinonasal diseases. It presents, both generic and distinct characteristics:

- *Soft tissue mass*: A well-defined soft tissue mass is often seen in the nasal cavity or paranasal sinuses.
- *Bone erosion*: In advanced cases, the tumor may invade and erode the surrounding bone, leading to bony destruction.
- *Sinus opacification*: The involved sinuses may appear opacified due to the presence of the tumor.
- *Focal hyperostosis*: mostly (74–90%), at the site of attachment two (**Figure 1**).

4.2 MRI

MRI is frequently recommended as the first imaging study because it provides excellent soft tissue contrast, enabling detailed visualization of the tumor's characteristic features, such as the convoluted cerebriform pattern.

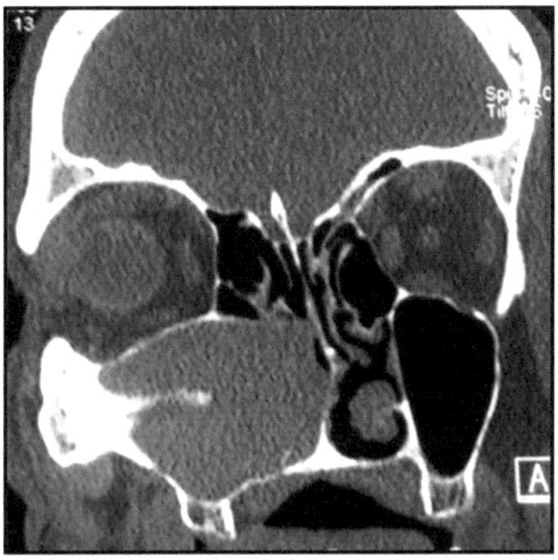

Figure 1.
CT of a maxillary IP.

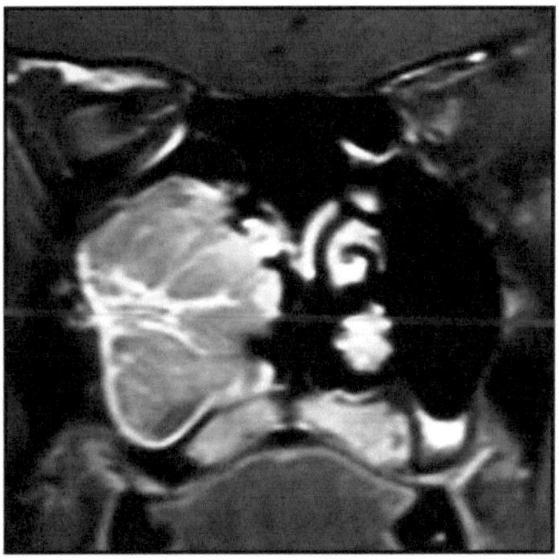

Figure 2.
MRI evaluation of the former patient.

- *Convoluted cerebriform pattern*: This is a highly characteristic finding on T2-weighted images. It appears as alternating bands of high and low signal intensity, resembling the gyri and sulci of the brain.

- *Contrast enhancement*: The tumor typically shows moderate to intense enhancement after the administration of contrast material (**Figure 2**).

4.3 Localization

IP primarily develops in the lateral nasal wall, particularly in the middle meatus region. The second most common location is the maxillary sinus, followed by the ethmoids. Involvement of the frontal and sphenoid sinuses is extremely rare and generally due to local extension from other sites. In a review of 1106 patients by Krouse in

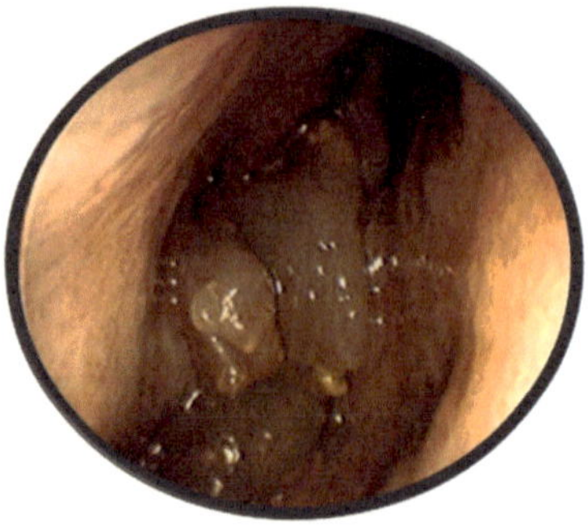

Figure 3.
Endoscopic appearance of a right maxillary IP, in the middle meatus.

2001, the lateral nasal wall was affected in 82% of cases, the maxillary sinus in 53.9%, the ethmoid in 31.6%, the frontal in 6.5%, and the sphenoid in 3.9% [4]. Nasal septum involvement was observed just in 9.9%. Intracranial invasion is rare and occurs most frequently through the cribriform plate or the roof of the ethmoid sinus, especially in recurrent lesions. In a recent paper, according to Budu et al., the maxillary and ethmoid sinuses were the most frequently involved sites, with simultaneous involvement occurring in 67.9% of cases. Isolated ethmoid sinus involvement was seen in 27.77% of cases. Involvement of the frontal and sphenoid sinuses was rare, with 1.85 and 2.46% of cases, respectively (**Figure 3**) [5].

4.4 Classifications

Various classification systems have been developed to categorize inverted papillomas (IP) based on their location and extent. These classifications aid surgeons in selecting the optimal surgical approach, determining the necessary extent of resection, and estimating the likelihood of recurrence. Krouse's and Han's systems are the most used, and they primarily consider the tumor's location and extent. However, more recent classifications, such as Kamel's system and Meng's system, focus on the tumor's origin within the nasal cavity and paranasal sinuses (**Table 1**) [5, 6].

Krouse staging system
Stage I disease is limited to the nasal cavity alone
Stage II disease is limited to the ethmoid sinuses and medial and superior portions of the maxillary sinuses
Stage III disease involves the lateral or inferior aspects of the maxillary sinuses or extension into the frontal or sphenoid sinuses
Stage IV disease involves any extra sinus involvement or all tumors with the concurrent malignant association

Table 1.
Krouse staging system.

4.5 Surgical principles

Surgery is considered the treatment of choice for inverted papilloma. Prior to the 1970s, IP was treated with a transnasal approach without microscopic or endoscopic assistance. This technique was associated with a high recurrence rate due to incomplete excision. Due to the limitations of the transnasal approach, medial maxillectomy with lateral rhinotomy was considered the gold standard until the 1980s [2, 3]. While more radical, this technique was associated with complications such as epiphora, chronic dacryocystitis, transient diplopia, and Eustachian tube dysfunction, and had potential esthetic sequelae due to external scars. To avoid these sequelae, surgical techniques without external incisions were introduced, such as the Rouge-Denker procedure, septal translocation, and midface degloving. The first report of endoscopic treatment of IP dates to 1981, when Stammberger documented 15 patients treated with an endoscopic approach. Since then, numerous authors have reported their experience in the endoscopic treatment of IP. Recurrence rates for the endoscopic versus non-endoscopic approach are described from 0% up to 34%, mainly from lesions with frontal sinus involvement, positive margins, sessile or multifocal attachments, and local dysplasia [7]. Over the years, transnasal endoscopic resection has become the standard of care in most cases, with external or combined approaches in selected patients. Histological studies of the attachment site of IPs prompt to underline that aggressive treatment of the latter has emerged as a key consideration in surgical planning to ensure complete tumor removal and minimize recurrence (**Figure 4**) [9].

So, the evolution in the endoscopic treatment of IPs, guided us to the principles of the *Pedicle oriented endoscopic surgery* (*POES*), as popularized in the last years. It enables tissue debulking with piecemeal resection (usually through a microdebrider), permitting a stepwise and meticulous removal of the tumor tissue, working toward the attachment site to minimize residual disease and surgical aggressiveness (**Figure 5**) [10, 11].

To achieve complete tumor removal and minimize recurrence, modern surgical approaches incorporate mucosal resection, subperiosteal dissection, and bone drilling or curettage at the tumor's attachment site (**Figure 6**).

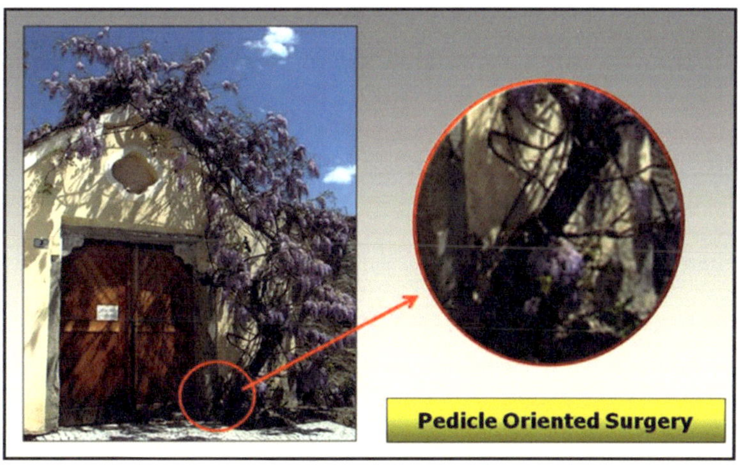

Figure 4.
Concept of the pedicle oriented endoscopic surgery [8].

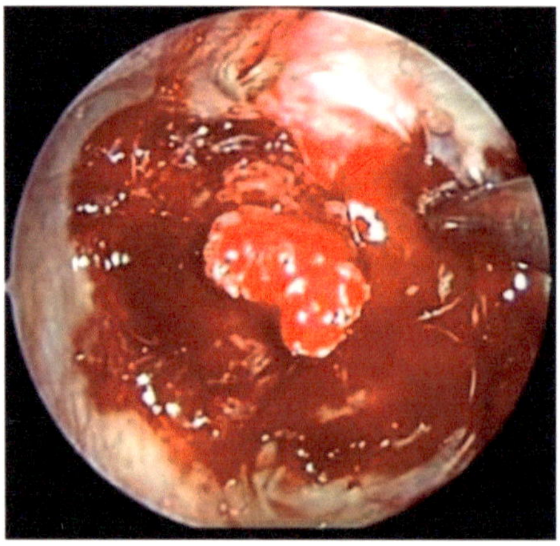

Figure 5.
Exposure of the site of attachment in the right maxillary sinus, during a POES procedure.

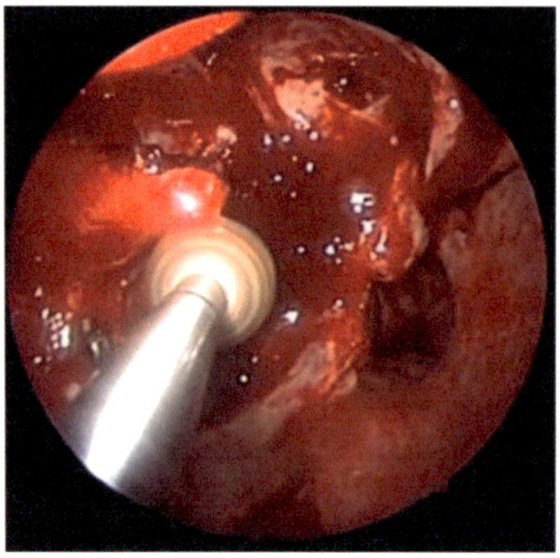

Figure 6.
Drilling of the former site of attachment.

Open or combined approaches (craniotomic, midfacial degloving, lateral rhinotomy), may still be necessary for complex cases involving most frequently the maxillary or frontal sinuses, for laterally attached tumors, ample recurrences and sessile or multicentric tumors [1, 12].

4.5.1 Surgical technique

Inverted papillomas limited to the nasal cavity and ethmoid, are generally easier to manage. However, those involving the maxillary, sphenoid, or frontal sinuses present sometimes a greater complexity. The extent of involvement within these sinuses and the precise attachment sites are critical factors in determining the optimal surgical strategy.

The introduction of advanced surgical tools, including microdebriders, angled scopes, and diamond drills, has revolutionized the endoscopic management of inverted papillomas. These tools allow precise tumor removal and bone work, especially in challenging locations like the skull base or laterally attached tumors. Additionally, neuronavigation (CT or MRI) may enhance surgical accuracy and safety in complex cases.

Whether the IP extends into the maxillary-sphenoid-frontal sinuses or originates within these sinuses, is a critical factor in determining the optimal surgical approach. Simple tumor extension can be treated through a middle meatotomy, sphenoidotomy, or frontal sinusotomy (generally a Draf II) [11].

A site of attachment within such sinuses presents a more complicated issue, that dictates special considerations in many cases.

4.5.2 Sphenoid sinus

IPs arising from the sphenoid sinus can typically be managed through a wide sphenoidotomy with the creation of a posterior septal window in some cases. This approach involves removing the anterior wall of the sphenoid sinus and often requires complete ethmoidectomy, to enhance visualization and surgical maneuverability.

Inverted papillomas arising from the lacerous-paraclival internal carotid artery (ICA) or optic canal, present two areas with the significant surgical challenges. Meticulous bone removal is necessary to ensure complete tumor excision without injuring these delicate structures [1, 13].

4.5.3 Maxillary sinus

Determining the precise wall(s) of the maxillary sinus to which the inverted papilloma is attached is essential for preoperative planning and optimizing the surgical approach.

Inverted papillomas that originate from the medial, posterior lateral, and superior walls of the maxillary sinus are generally easier to treat. On the other hand, those arising from the anterior and inferior walls are more complex to manage and have a higher likelihood of recurrence; moreover, areas such as the prelacrimal and alveolar recesses, are generally tricky to manage.

The transnasal endoscopic medial maxillectomy (EMM) was first introduced in 1995 with many subsequent variations, that point to dominate the most anterior and inferior areas of the sinus, extended (EEMM) or not the anterior part of the inferior turbinate and the nasolacrimal duct (NLD) [7, 10, 14]. Eventual extension to the pyriform aperture codifies the Endoscopic Denker or Sturman-Canfield approach to reach the outmost anterior or far lateral wall [15].

The application of the POES strategy led to the development of several pedicle oriented endoscopic modules for the treatment of maxillary IPs, namely Pedicle Oriented Endoscopic Meatotomy (POEM), Pedicle Oriented Endoscopic Middle Maxillectomy (POEMM), and Pedicle Oriented Endoscopic Extended Middle Maxillectomy (POEEMM), which differ in the extent of resection.

The key difference between POEMs (POEM, POEMM, POEEMM) and other classical maxillectomies (MME, MMEA) is that the tumor gets debulked in a centripetal direction, but the mucoperiosteum removal and bone drilling, regard a peri-tumoral area and not the entire surgical field [10].

Transseptal approaches have been proposed too, that facilitate access and a three or four hands technique for anterior or inferior IPs in the maxillary sinus [16].

Most recently, Zhou et al. presented the prelacrimal recess approach (PLA), which provides excellent access to all walls of the maxillary sinus, including the prelacrimal and alveolar recesses, while preserving the inferior turbinate and nasal lateral wall [17]. The PLA can be extended anteriorly to the pyriform aperture or converted to a standard endoscopic medial maxillectomy [18, 19]. Based on the same concept a reversible endoscopic medial maxillectomy approach was presented; in that case, the entire lateral nasal wall is displaced medially for tumor resection and replaced at the end of the procedure [20, 21].

4.5.4 Frontal sinus

Surgery depends on the individual patient's anatomy, specific site of attachment, and extent of the mass. IPs originating from the nasal cavity/ethmoid and extending into the frontal sinus can typically be removed through the frontal sinus ostium, with a frontal sinusotomy (Draf I, Draf IIa, IIb, or Draf III). Inverted papillomas that arise within the frontal sinus necessitate specific surgical approaches due to their complex anatomy and potential for difficult access. Precise identification of the tumor's attachment site is very important. Most lesions may be treated through a frontal sinusotomy (Draf II a-b) with or without a septal window and contralateral access or a Draf III, with the concomitant use of angled scopes and drills [22]. Tumors located far laterally may require additional endoscopic surgical techniques, or osteoplastic flaps, alone or in combination. Between the former, the orbital transposition approach and, more recently, the periorbital suspension approach was introduced to deal with lateral and/or superior frontal sinus lesions [17, 23]. Among the later, usual indications are extensive frontal recurrence, impossibility to endoscopic exposure (in particular, anterior wall), and multifocal disease [1, 24]. Extensive involvement of the anterior/posterior walls, extension into the intracranial or subcutaneous space, or dysplasia/carcinoma, may require traditional transcranial approaches such as a classic craniofacial resection.

4.5.5 Recurrence rate

The primary risk factor for the recurrence of IP is an incomplete surgical resection. Factors such as involvement of the frontal sinus, sessile growth patterns, positive tumor margins, multifocal disease, and the presence of dysplasia are associated with a higher risk of recurrence. Recurrences usually present within 2 years postoperatively, and, generally, recurrences during the first post-op year should be considered residual tumors [1–3]. Recurrences according to Krouse's system, were stated at around 0% in T1 stage, 16% in T2 stage, 25% in T3 stage, and 60% in T4 stage, in a recent report [25].

4.5.6 IP and associated malignancy

The most common malignant neoplasm associated with inverted papilloma (IP) is undoubtedly squamous cell carcinoma (SCC). Several types of associations between IP and SCC have been described:

1. Synchronous carcinoma within IP.

2. Areas of carcinoma in situ within IP.

3. Areas of IP within SCC.

4. Metachronous SCC not associated with the original site of the IP.

5. Metachronous SCC at the original site of the IP, otherwise known as "malignant transformation.

HPV types 6/11 and 16/18 have been linked to inverted papillomas with severe dysplasia and squamous cell carcinoma, suggesting a potential role in malignant transformation [26, 27]. The risk of malignant transformation is estimated around 5–15% of cases.

In such cases disease staging becomes imperative, eventual multidisciplinary evaluation is advised, and in most cases, surgery with adjuvant therapy is recommended.

5. Conclusion

Inverted papilloma (IP) is a benign tumor with a variable biological behavior. Its propensity for local invasion, difficulty in identifying the precise origin, high recurrence rate, and potential for malignant transformation make it a challenging clinical entity. While the exact etiology remains elusive, evidence suggests a role for human papillomavirus (HPV) DNA in recurrence and malignant transformation.

Complete surgical resection remains the cornerstone of treatment. Endoscopic techniques, such as endoscopic sinus surgery (ESS), have become the standard approach for most cases, offering minimal invasiveness and good outcomes. For more complex cases involving the maxillary sinus or frontal sinus, techniques like medial maxillectomy or extended endoscopic sinus surgery may be necessary. In rare instances, traditional open surgical approaches may be required for extensive or recurrent disease.

Long-term follow-up is highly recommended with adjunctive MRI examination in the first 2 years and in case of suspected lesions.

Author details

Georgios Giourgos
ORL Clinic, ASST Papa Giovanni XXIII, Bergamo, Italy

*Address all correspondence to: ggdoc1@yahoo.com

References

[1] Kamel RH, Khaled A, Abdelfattah AF, et al. Surgical treatment of sinonasal inverted papilloma. Current Opinion in Otolaryngology & Head and Neck Surgery. 2022;**30**(1):26-32

[2] Lund VJ, Stammberger H, Nicolai P, et al. European position paper on endoscopic management of tumours of the nose, paranasal sinuses and skull base. Rhinology. Supplement. 2010;**22**:1-143

[3] Lawson W, Kaufman MR, Biller HF. Treatment outcomes in the management of inverted papilloma: An analysis of 160 cases. Laryngoscope. 2003;**113**:1548-1556

[4] Krouse JH. Development of a staging system for inverted papilloma. Laryngoscope. 2000;**110**:965-968

[5] Budu V, Schnaider A, Bulescu I. Endoscopic approach of sinonasal inverted papilloma—Our 15 years' experience on 162 cases. Romanian Journal of Rhinology. 2015;**5**(17):31-36

[6] Han JK, Smith TL, Loehrl T, et al. An evolution in the management of sinonasal inverting papilloma. Laryngoscope. 2001;**111**:1395-1400

[7] Kamel R, Khaled A, Kandil T. Inverted papilloma: New classification and guidelines for endoscopic surgery. American Journal of Rhinology. 2005;**19**:358-364

[8] Giourgos G. Chirurgia endoscopica del peduncolo nel Papilloma invertito mascellare: Il concetto della POES e l'applicazione alla localizzazione mascellare (Italian Edition). In: Edizioni Accademiche Italiane, editor. 2019

[9] Wang Y, An Y, Zhao C, et al. Attachment-oriented endoscopic treatment of inverted papilloma involving the frontal sinus/recess. The Journal of Craniofacial Surgery. 2020;**31**:e778-e781

[10] Pagella F, Pusateri A, Giourgos G, et al. Evolution in the treatment of sinonasal inverted papilloma: Pedicle-oriented endoscopic surgery. American Journal of Rhinology & Allergy. 2014;**28**:75-81

[11] Pagella F, Giourgos G, Matti E, et al. Endoscopic treatment of maxillary inverted papilloma. Rhinology. 2011;**49**:369-374

[12] Ferrari M, Schreiber A, Mattavelli D, et al. How aggressive should resection of inverted papilloma be? Refinement of surgical planning based on the 25-year experience of a single tertiary center. International Forum of Allergy & Rhinology. 2020;**10**:619-628

[13] Coutinho G, Marques J, Leal M, et al. Surgical outcomes of sinonasal inverted papilloma: A 17 year review. Brazilian Journal of Otorhinolaryngology. 2020;**86**:315-320

[14] Kamel RH. Transnasal endoscopic medial maxillectomy in inverted papilloma. Laryngoscope. 1995;**105**:847-853

[15] Stavrakas M, Karkos PD, Tsinaslanidou Z, Constantinidis J. Endoscopic Denker's approach for the treatment of extensive sinonasal tumors: Our experience. Laryngoscope. 2021;**131**:1458-1462

[16] Omura K, Nomura K, Aoki S, et al. Resection of inverted papilloma in nasal cavity with transseptal

access and crossing multiple incisions minimizes bleeding and reveals the tumor pedicle. Auris Nasus Larynx. 2020;**47**:410-414

[17] Karligkiotis A, Pistochini A, Turri-Zanoni M, et al. Endoscopic endonasal orbital transposition to expand the frontal sinus approaches. American Journal of Rhinology & Allergy. 2015;**29**(6):449-456

[18] Arosio AD, Valentini M, Canevari FR, et al. Endoscopic endonasal prelacrimal approach: Radiological considerations, morbidity, and outcomes. Laryngoscope. 2021;**131**:1715-1721

[19] Lee JT, Yoo F, Wang M, et al. Modified endoscopic Denker approach in management of inverted papilloma of the anterior maxillary sinus. International Forum of Allergy and Rhinology. 2020;**10**:533-538

[20] Tepedino MS, Ferrão ACM, Higa HCM, et al. Reversible endoscopic medial maxillectomy: Endonasal approach to diseases of the maxillary sinus. International Archives of Otorhinolaryngology. 2020;**24**(2): e247-e252

[21] Zhou B, Han DM, Cui SJ, et al. Endoscopic nasal lateral wall dissection approach to maxillary sinus. Zhonghua Er Bi Yan Hou Tou JingWai Ke Za Zhi. 2007;**42**:743-748

[22] Pietrobon G, Karligkiotis A, Turri-Zanoni M, et al. Surgical management of inverted papilloma involving the frontal sinus: A practical algorithm for treatment planning. Acta Otorhinolaryngologica Italica. 2019;**39**:28-39

[23] Tilak A, Purvis J, Peña-Garcia A, et al. Above and beyond: Periorbital suspension for endoscopic access to difficult frontal sinus pathology. Laryngoscope. Mar 2022;**132**(3):538-544

[24] Sham CL, van Hasselt CA, Chow SMW, et al. Frontal inverted papillomas: A 25-year study. Laryngoscope. 2019;**130**:1622-1628

[25] Makihara S, Kariya S, Naito T, et al. Attachment-oriented endoscopic surgical management for inverted papillomas in the nasal cavity and paranasal sinuses. Auris Nasus Larynx. 2019;**46**:748-753

[26] Contrera KJ, Woody NM, Rahman M, et al. Clinical management of emerging sinonasal malignancies. Head & Neck. 2020;**42**:2202-2212

[27] Kamath MP, Shenoy SV, Prasad V, Bhojwani K, Pai R, Mathew NM. Inverted papilloma of atypical origin with unusual extension into the oropharynx. Journal of Cancer Research and Therapeutics. 2015;**11**(3):666